PENGUIN BOOKS

I0459677

TETHERED

Tracy was at the start of her law career and at the cusp of life when she got a debilitating brainstem stroke that affected her speech, eyesight, and ability to breathe and swallow. It also severely weakened her left side and completely paralysed her right. She found herself, effectively, a thinking statue at the age of thirty-five.

This is an account of her journey to recovery. As her brain is reset, she finds, so is her life. Like a growing child, she learns the most basic things anew, and more insightfully, the second time around. She sees the world in a different dimension this time—as wheelchair-bound. She discovers what faith means when it is all that is left.

In amusing and heart-wrenching anecdotes, she finds that there is a life to be had, even in the cracks.

Tethered

Tracy Anne Ong

PENGUIN BOOKS

An imprint of Penguin Random House

PENGUIN BOOKS

Penguin Books is an imprint of the Penguin Random House group of
companies whose addresses can be found at
global.penguinrandomhouse.com

Published by Penguin Random House SEA Pte Ltd
40 Penjuru Lane, #03-12, Block 2
Singapore 609216

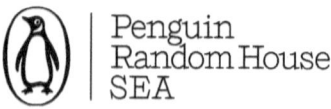

First published in Penguin Books by Penguin Random House SEA 2024

ISBN 9789815127904

Typeset in Garamond by MAP Systems, Bengaluru, India

www.penguin.sg

To my family

'I have on my table a violin string. It is free to move in any direction I like. If I twist it, it responds; it is free. But it is not free to sing. So I take it and fix it into my violin. I bind it and when it is bound, it is free for the first time to sing.'

—Rabindranath Tagore

Author's Note

I wrote vignettes of my illness while I was experiencing it. Everything then was in the present tense. Slowly, I found them as events in the past as I steadily hurdled them. Fast forward to now, more than two years later, and you are holding this book.

I've changed the names and identifying details of some people whose stories I tell, but I am grateful to all of them who make up my story.

Prologue

My brain is my biggest boon and biggest bane. When I was thirty-five, part of my brain stopped working on me. I had a dissection of my vertebra-basilar arteries, leading to a brainstem stroke that affected my breathing, swallowing, speech, eyesight, and severely weakened my left and paralysed my right. It was explained to me as the tearing of a superhighway that each held specific functions. Once my arteries tore, it left a site of mass destruction, of rubble and forever-altered lives without an ending. I could only breathe a deep sigh of relief that some parts of the superhighway somehow missed the great earthquake that swallowed me whole and spat me out.

This is not a depressing book, but it is an account that begins with immense suffering. Suffering that demands every bit of you. A suffering that purges the soul. So, I hope you will not be taken aback by this beginning, for as with all things, this is only the beginning.

Part 1

1

19 March 2022, Philippines

It started innocently enough. I was chatting with my mom and sister when I felt a subtle shutting off behind my eyes. It was so subtle. It only felt like a flicker, not even a blackout, but I knew something was wrong, like a wire had tripped.

I lay down on the couch thinking I had the stomach flu from the shellfish I ate the day before. It felt as mundane as that—like I had a bloated stomach, that food was floating within me. When the feeling didn't let up, I walked to my room to rest, but mid-way, I puked. I felt well enough to climb up the steps to my second-floor bedroom to take a nap.

I vomited ten more times that afternoon. After vomiting, my eyes would stabilize for a few minutes, allowing me to wash my face and take a leak, but then it would start again—that floaty feeling. Like being on a boat or on your tiptoes for too long a time. Just as quietly as the feeling would leave, it would come back again. There was a tingling feeling bubbling up in my left limbs, but it was mild, and I chalked it up to dehydration. When I was losing too much fluid, my family decided to take me to the hospital Emergency Room. I'll always remember what I had the last time in the house, when I had not a care in the world, except the ordinary cares of an uneventful passing Saturday, made a little unfortunate by diarrhoea—sweet potatoes and saltine crackers. It would be the last careless meal I'd have for a very long time.

2

I flailed down the steps as I got myself into the car that would take me to the ER. For some unknown reason, my eyes seemed to be playing tricks on me, and I couldn't keep my balance. Around 9.30 p.m., we arrived at the ER. I clambered out of the car, thinking that my legs could still hold me. I would have fallen, if not for the security guard who hurriedly shoved a wheelchair to catch me. By then, my legs had turned to jelly.

As in all third-world countries, there was a queue at the ER. I watched as someone with heart disease or someone suspected positive for COVID-19 was rushed in before me. We patiently waited for our turn, as the cool air billowed in the night sky. There was a mom carrying her baby, suffering from a fever. We were the fourth or fifth in line.

Our turn finally came. A resident took my stats and ran down a checklist to make sure I did not have COVID-19. Back then, the ER was still divided between the COVID-19 and non-COVID-19 wards. They opened an isolated room for me, as barely three months ago, I was found to have an auto-immune disease. They took my age, height, and weight. It would be the fullness of what I would be for the next months. I would be reduced to paper and referred to as a bed number. Thirty-five, five feet one inch, and sixty-one kilos. The whole of my life, vibrant and throbbing, reduced to impersonal statistics near the end. When push comes to shove, we shudder to think of what we are when frozen in time.

But of course, I didn't have these thoughts then. I was just being admitted.

3

The ceiling was grey. The air was cold in that small room we were stowed away in. It had its own restroom, for which I was eternally grateful, and two plastic chairs to billet us in. It was like a utility room turned isolation room, but it felt like such a privilege then.

It was there that I found that I could no longer swallow. It seems unfathomable to have something so expected and normal wrenched from you, but try as I might, I could not feel any sensation of swallowing. It was like saliva going down a black hole. I tried to shove it down my throat, but I couldn't feel it once it was down there. There was none of the familiar clicking sound that told you the food you spooned in was going successfully down the throat. It was alarming to say the least. It was like speaking and being met with deafening silence. Silence that wasn't supposed to be there.

Panicked, we alerted the nurses of the new development. The resident came in with a bottle of water for me to sip. *Had I really lost my ability to swallow forever? Or did my body still remember what my brain couldn't?* Thankfully, my throat muscles remembered to close as I sipped the water. I sipped the water unknowing what would happen. It was the beginning of a lot of unknowing. What was clear was that the degeneration was progressing, and I was in the thick of it.

I had my COVID-19 test done about four hours after I arrived. I couldn't have any other tests done on me until I tested negative for the virus. We had no idea why we had to wait so long for this test that allowed me to take more consequential ones. *Could we not have had it faster at a drive-through?* It was mind-boggling. I remember my sister, Kim, begging desperately that I have it sooner, but we'd soon find that there is no place for pleading in a hospital. The more expensive, speedier test would yield results four hours later.

The morning broke our senseless waiting. I had my MRI done just when the sun was rising. Kim and my dad had been seated in plastic chairs outside for eight hours now. *They could have gotten a full night of sleep out there.* The MRI technician who met us said his team was waiting all night for a patient. I was exhausted, having stayed awake all night. I slept soundly at the start of every round of noisy hammering from the machine. My breathing melded well with the drilling of the machine that was scanning my brain. I was glad I could take a rest in the most uneasy of circumstances. The machine seemed like a bulky, enveloping friend. I drifted off to a deep sleep.

4

I breathed a sigh of relief as the resident came in with news that my MRI scan was clear. A weight was lifted from the air. Though the hospital was an unfriendly place to some people, it had always been kind to me. The downside of the news was that they didn't know what was wrong with me. My team of doctors subjected me to a series of tests—ultrasounds, nerve tests, etc. They poked needle after needle in my veins until they were bruised and blue, and there was no good vein left to poke. I cleared all the exams, but by then the whole left side of my body was paralysed. I was in a quandary, and it felt safer then to not know than to know.

5

That afternoon, I decided to take things in my own hands. I was afraid my hair was getting too oily from everyone caressing it. We were told only ICU nurses gave baths, so being in the ward, I figured we had to do it ourselves. My mom spread out an absorbent pad around my hair and used a plastic bowl as a basin upon which to wash my hair with cups of water. I rested my neck at the edge of the bowl. It was uncomfortable and jarring on my neck.

I always look back at that moment. *Did I extend my neck too soon too much over a mundane care as to forever change my life?* I ask because after that I felt a noticeable headache spread throughout my head. I asked my doctor for medicine, and she gave me a painkiller that made me drift off to my last good sleep for four hours. When the painkiller wore away, the pain grew back. Shortly thereafter, the tingles that spread slowly but steadily on my left spread rapidly on my right. It was a tingling that came with muscle weakness, like creeping ants slowly but surely eating the life out of me. Soon after, I felt the muscles on the left side of my face start to droop. My speech noticeably slurred. The evolving nature of whatever disease was plaguing me was already undeniable.

We alerted the resident. Despite my palsy and the sudden onslaught of symptoms, she told me not to worry, that I was already on stroke medication. My neurologist had put me on stroke medication while figuring out what my exact disease was. It was nearing midnight, and there was nothing more that they could do.

We should wait until morning. I lay resigned and unargumentative on my bed. They were the doctors. My life was in their hands.

I was unusually calm that night, like a very level-headed version of myself took over. Sensing that I was losing control over my right as the tingling slowly took over the right side of my body, I hastily wrote in jagged handwriting all the usernames and passcodes of the bank accounts and emails I handled on the back of a used brown envelope. My handwriting, though crooked, was still legible. I will forever thank that girl who took over, for her foresight and equanimity at the mouth of debilitating change, for soon after, both left and right parts of my body were effectively paralysed.

6

The next morning, they hurried me in a stretcher to the MRI room. By then, I had difficulty swallowing my own sputum which made me hesitant to lie on my back in a white tunnel for a considerable amount of time with dye running through my veins. No nurse would be able to suction out my sputum while under the machine. I urged my family and the technicians on with my eyes, as they conversed before me, as if to say to get on it before the saliva started pooling. I didn't want to open my mouth to say anything, afraid that saliva would flow down the wrong tube. Finally, they had everything sorted out, and it was all systems go for me. My left hand was too weak to press the emergency button so I should just wiggle my left foot, which still had slight movement, in case I needed something.

The MRI yielded a sigh of relief. The news of a stroke never came so welcome. Finally, we knew what was wrong with me. My neurologist in the Philippines was suspicious it was between a stroke or Guillain-Barré syndrome (GBS). GBS starts with a tingling feeling in the legs like pins and needles that spreads rapidly to paralysis. I was shoved between a rock and a hard place, but at least I knew now what I had.

I waited patiently as the people surrounding me struggled to find me a room in the ICU. I do not think I fully grasped the blow that I was dealt with because I was preoccupied with the little things, like how to pee in a bedpan with my pants stripped down.

It was either that, or I had so much faith that medicine could save me. But I was terribly wrong that time.

By ambulance, I was transferred on a stretcher to an older branch of the hospital. My father accompanied me on the ride. I could see the bright lights of the city and could hear the noisy siren of the ambulance. It seemed quite desperate to find myself in an ambulance being the rider, being the patient. I had so often given way to one, never thinking I would be given way.

I felt relieved and happy to arrive in my room in the ICU. Finally, I could have my own clean bed, get washed up, and catch peaceful sleep after the clutter of the day. I let myself be positioned comfortably on the bed before I drifted off to a dreamless sleep. I woke up after several hours, complaining that my back hurt. The nurse came in to reposition me. Such a mundane care from me—that my back hurt—but it all went downhill from there.

7

It seemed like a time vacuum, but things progressed quickly after that. My speech slurred until it disappeared completely. My tongue retreated to its cave. I jerked uncontrollably, like being possessed of intermittent seizures. I was told to wear high-cut sneakers to prevent foot drop and compression stockings to keep my blood flowing. My left eyelid would not clasp shut. I lost eye control. I became cross-eyed and had double vision. I used letters on a communication board to spell out what I wanted to say. Because my eyes were seeing two images separately, I couldn't point to the exact letters I wanted, leaving everyone to guess which letters I meant exactly. It exasperated me when my family did not get what I wanted to say. I resigned myself to many things that I couldn't have because I couldn't ask for them. If I felt uncomfortable, I stayed that way because I could not express what I wanted. A little scratch here and there would be too nuanced to ask for. Beggars could not be choosers.

Anticipating my decline, I calmly gestured to Kim that one blink meant yes, and two blinks meant no. I thought I blinked both eyes, but my left eye remained stark open. I could not move all my four limbs any more and could only manage a thumbs-up. I was unusually calm for someone who had anticipated her degeneration. Maybe we are wired that way, that there's this back-up program that runs when we're falling apart. The previous day, I had told my mom and dad that if I could no longer speak,

I wanted them to know that I love them and thank them for everything. I was covering all my bases.

Medical staff came in to perform tests on me. Kim spoke of adventures we had yet to go on. *Did I want to go to Berkeley and study again? Did I want to go to the Dolomites or Patagonia?* She went all out. One blink. Two blinks. It's funny how when life rushes near death, you want none of it.

It was like a checklist. I had to get my catheter and nasogastric tube (NGT) inserted before I was too weak for them to attach it. I had given myself up willingly to machines to support me. Inserting a catheter required me to spread open my legs while a bunch of residents and interns gathered around to attach a tube to my urethra. It was like a series of embarrassments I had to go through; people assumed I automatically shed all my cares when I got sick. By necessity, it had to be done as quietly and smoothly as they needed it in. I had to relax as they inserted the NGT down my nose and throat. They said it was going to be very uncomfortable. I picked the nostril they were to insert the tube in. I had nasal allergies in one nostril, so I opted for them to insert it in my right one.

I remember when my grandmother was sick, it took a while for her to eat through a tube. But in a matter of a day in the ICU, I had to be on one. I was fully aware of where my grandmother's condition had led her. If I were going there, I needed her to be with me.

8

I don't know when I needed oxygen support, but it soon came. I don't remember it being installed. I just remember sucking in clean air from the tubes until the very end of them, when phlegm seemed to clog the tubes that connected me to life.

I don't know exactly when I partly lost my consciousness. I could keep track of the dates. I heard everything around me. But upon looking back, I am not exactly sure I know all that happened in that dark room. I don't know when I lost my voice, nor when I started seeing double. Such a panic as I assumed would come never swept over me. I don't remember myself reacting. It was like knowing something but not understanding.

They put me on maximum steroids. It was supposed to be a wonder drug. They put me on one gram per day, and this put my dreams into hyperdrive. I dreamt that my relatives were having a Korean dinner beside my bed, with a full spread laid out. Only, the guest of honour was late, and nobody could touch the food. I dreamt that I had drafted a legal contract, and since I couldn't move, I needed help from my sisters to print it. I dreamt of how to repay my nurses. I dreamt that each letter in the alphabet bore a challenge that I had to hurdle, and I was stuck on the letter F. I knew how to get past it. I only had to make the fully conscious people know it. '*Remove me from Farrington*,' I pleaded. The dream was so vivid that it was a narrative I lived in even while I was awake. The plot was so real to me that I was frustrated when my watcher couldn't get me. I asked my sisters to call my two kid cousins to see whether they could get me out of Farrington. Maybe their childhood eyes could see the supermarket named Farrington I was trapped in. I didn't know how they could get me out. But I wanted them to code me out. I felt trapped in a game, and I so desperately wanted out. My sisters feared I was losing my mind. Out of desperation, they asked my neurologist if she knew what Farrington was.

The worst dreams were when I'd wake, forgetting I couldn't breathe and move easily. My brainstem stroke affected the primitive features of my brain, including breathing and motor control. There were nights when I was running in a field of wildflowers with my hands grazing the top of the blades of grass. Then I'd wake up; the dream would come to a screeching halt with me gasping for air. I wanted to run through the field of my dreams, but I was trapped in my immobile body. I told my sisters to move my legs every two hours. They felt like concrete logs attached to my body. I thought about rigor mortis. Is that why our limbs automatically stiffen upon death? Is it because they've suddenly lost a command centre?

When you are going downhill, and you're sliding down fast, your reaction time is not fast enough to realize how far down you have gone. Soon enough, I couldn't carry my own head. It would fling violently to the sides as I would be turned to be cleaned and wiped down. Now I understand why they prize having a good head on your shoulders. I couldn't keep mine on my own if I wanted to.

One night, I struggled to buy my mom and sister cranberry muffins at a Starbucks. I couldn't lift my leg, but I tried my best to make the short distance to the cashier. Somehow, I was convinced that I had taken the muffins back to the hospital, and it was right on the table beside me. Of course, it was a dream, but I woke up having slight movement in my left leg and arm. I kept moving my arm until I could make a wobbly fist in the air. I kept sliding my left leg up and down the bed, intent on bringing out what little movement had come back for good.

As I sprung my fist into the air, I noticed how I couldn't interlock my thumb and index finger as I could just moments ago. I assessed and reassessed. I didn't want to raise a false alarm. I kept moving my fingers. *A co-ordination problem*, I thought. I was losing my co-ordination.

I alerted the nurse. She scheduled me for an MRI the next morning. She probably could read the concern in my eyes. She called up technicians from the other hospital to conduct an MRI scan on me 'stat'.

There was no new stroke, the neurologist assured me. A new stroke would have painted a new light colour in the MRI scan, but mine only showed that any sign of stroke was dulling, and therefore, my brain was recovering. Reassured, I drifted to a long sleep.

It all seems fast-paced now because of the big events that bombarded us, but time was as slow as a snail's pace then. I used to stare into my mother's eyes, conveying desperately, *how in the world am I to survive the next day?* The waiting while almost completely immobile was painful. Time hung in the air with no end in sight. No resolution at the end of a tunnel. It was a straddling, and I felt every silent minute of it.

I looked at my mother and thought how terrible it was that she should witness her child have a stroke in her lifetime. She was greyed and thin from her mother's passing a couple of months ago. She had barely recovered, and now this. It was the first time that I cried, seeing my pain mirrored in her eyes. It was a pain that couldn't be avoided. Tears sprang from my right eye. The left side of my face was frozen. Somehow my brain couldn't command my left eye to cry.

I glanced at my father behind the glass doors of the ICU. I hardly glanced his way in a day, but he stayed seated in a plastic chair outside my door from morning until evening. He would have nothing to do but stare at me, toy listlessly with his phone, and run errands outside for needs I had. He could not come in the ICU like the rest of the family because I couldn't risk being exposed to people who had contact with the outside world.

Kim pasted sticky get well notes from my loved ones on the wall and hung blue and silver *banderitas* on my birthday. She would dreamily scroll through pictures of Italian homes with me for us to renovate together if I got better; this was before my eyesight drastically deteriorated. A nurse said Kim knelt and prayed as I slept in the ICU. I felt her crying, desperately wanting me to get better. *How do you submit to the will of God when you so desperately want an outcome?* Her hurting was palpable.

My youngest sister, Mimi, a doctor, wrote to researchers who wrote about the most unique of diseases in medical journals to get an understanding of my case. One was even nice enough to answer. I imagine it must be hard being the only doctor in the family, answering all questions without a definite answer at that time.

My birthday came and passed. Holy Week started. A storm came. Doctors went on vacation. Interns came to do their routine tests repeatedly. No matter how hard I tried to keep track of the time, I lost count of the days. The days were as bleak as the dark clouds that hovered over the roof deck of the old building I could see by my window. The days were as static as the scene frozen in the picture frame hanging on my wall—as if in abeyance for I did not know what. I filled my days with food and hiking videos Kim downloaded for me in a USB. Nurses came in to prick my finger before pouring milk down my tube. They jabbed at my abdomen to thin my blood. My abdomen was violet and green with bruises. My urine in my catheter was coloured the shade of my blood. My catheter had to be removed and reinserted—to my utter embarrassment and discomfort—regularly to prevent infections. Chest X-ray technicians came to wake me up at dawn and Cough Assists tried to make me cough to no avail. Medical technicians patted at my back, cupping their hands over my shoulders to make breathing easier. I was nebulized several times a day to loosen any phlegm that may have stuck stubbornly to my back. They regularly probed my throat for any saliva that may have collected in it (because I could not swallow it) with a suction tube until the abrasiveness of the whole exercise would make me choke the tube out breathlessly. My intravenous cannula had to be reinserted every time it was dislodged or no longer patent until I had no good vein left. My hand was black and blue. They drew blood from me at odd hours and sent them to more advanced cities for study. Everything was a routine of procedures I was getting used to.

Sleeping was the hard part. I dreaded it the most. Because of the steroids, I found my brain almost impossible to dull to sleep. It was supercharged. We tried evening meditation. Eventually, I settled on Mimi reading me a very boring book to sleep. I concentrated on her quiet monotone voice against the quiet hum of the air conditioner and let it make me drift off to sleep. I would dip in and out of the acceptable vital statistics in the ICU monitor. I vaguely remember a nurse commiserating in my dream-filled sleep one of the nights, staying with me in the room.

Then day would dawn, bringing the same stories all over again. I would let all hope drain from my eyes. I just wanted to sleep through it all. Not long after, I soon found a rhythm. Every couple of hours, I would be turned on my opposite side, and as soon as the nurse would prop my leg on the pillow, I would will myself to sleep. I didn't want to be woken for my doctors, save for this sweet-voiced doctor who always came early. All they ever seemed to do was wake me up and tell me what I already knew. They seemed to be never there when I needed them at the critical times.[1]

---

[1] I want to stress that this was how I felt and had nothing to do with how they actually treated me.

Day-in and day-out, I would see other beds being wheeled out of the ICU in a gurney either to transfer to the general ward or the morgue. By the window of my room, I witnessed heart patients being rushed back to the operating room across mine to have their chests reopened after having just survived a surgery. It was a very gloomy environment I lived in. Every afternoon, the sun would stream in to cast an almost sickly sepia glow in my room. I could not stand it. I found it easier to draw the curtains and lose count of the days.

In the thickest of these dark days, I was conscious of two angels standing in my room. One was by the door standing guard. He had a suit of heavy armour on. The other was by my bedside, white and feathery. They were mostly stationary, but I felt one by my bed distinctly holding me, my chest particularly, as if keeping me from falling, as if holding me up. I couldn't see their faces clearly, just the faint outline of them. I didn't make much of them. They were like my silent companions for a couple of days. I didn't find the urge or the fancy to tell anyone about them until the weekend when I pointed unsteadily at the communication board, *I saw the helpers of God.* I don't know why I didn't call them angels. It elicited such wonder among my mom and Kim that I wondered why I had not thought much of it before. I was mad at God, mad at his angels for just staring and holding me while I was wasting away and struggling for my life. Was He not known for His saving power? I needed Him to save me, yet I felt forsaken by Him.

Looking back, Kim says I started getting better from that moment. Though my eyes were seeing double, they dilated my eyes and found nothing troubling there. They did several chest X-rays on me, and somehow no phlegm ever went past my throat. They dropped a metal ball down my throat and found that my vocal cords were perfectly well. True enough, one day in the midst of watching travel videos, I uttered the name of the show that was playing on YouTube. 'SOHO,' I muttered, saying the name of the host with a brokenness, but an utterance, nonetheless. I talked and talked then, making friends out of my nurses. In my mind, I was speaking our dialect smoothly, but to my listener, it was like a sound coming out of frozen lips.

I didn't know what my angelic visitors' touch meant. Later in the hospital, I would find the verse that mirrored my experience and shuddered that they did exactly to me as promised. 'For He will order His angels to protect you wherever you go. They will hold you up with their hands so you won't even hurt your feet on the stone.' (Psalm 91:11-12, NLT)

Everything may have been blurry then, but all I know is I would have no motivation to make up stories for myself in that state. If they were hallucinations, they were what I hallucinated about at a time when I didn't want anything to do with them. I saw everything in double, but there was just distinctly one of each of them. In whatever level of consciousness they may have come, I turned a corner from then on.

9

They brought in a speech therapist from the outside. The hospital didn't have one in their ranks. For some reason, they had to sneak her in, as if the hospital had the monopoly to cure me. She began asking me background questions that made me utter sounds she wanted to hear. How old I was. Where I lived. What I did before I had the stroke.

The last question got to me. I hadn't had the chance to mourn myself. Somehow in all the hullabaloo, I forgot to. It's amazing how one event in your life can scrap who you were. Like in the whoosh of an eraser, your past is erased. Who you were becomes irrelevant. 'A lawyer,' I said in between tears. I thought I said the word, but my mouth barely moved.

The speech therapist made me read through vowels and syllables, trying to make my mouth form the shapes that make the sounds. My mouth could barely form a pout. My tongue could hardly come out of its cave. My pitch was terrible. My voice stayed in a high register. One day, to tickle my swallowing muscles, she dredged a cotton bud in lemon juice and put it in my mouth. It threw me into a coughing fit. Residents were called to my room. My mom and I bet she got a scare. *Did it go down the wrong tube?*

Occupational and physical therapists also visited me. Sometimes they came; sometimes they didn't. On the days they came, they would prop my head on a strategically folded towel to hold it in place and pull passively on my legs and arms. They would place a popsicle stick a short distance from my lips so I would have to extend out my tongue to reach it. They would pretend the popsicle stick was my favourite ice drop. Periodically, I would spew out thick, green phlegm. Often times, it would land on their scrubs. I would apologetically look at them. I had no choice; I had to dislodge the phlegm in my chest in order to breathe. The physical therapists and the nurses would hoist me up, three people at a time, so I could sit up on my bed for a few seconds to dangle my legs. My back would feel incredibly heavy, like a load of cement bricks. I could only sit myself up for a few seconds at a time. They would tie my hands with an elastic bandage to rotating hand pedals, so my hands would not slip out of them. I could no longer grasp at things; I had no control over my fingers. Suddenly, they were these flailing useless things.

I had a myriad of doctors working with me, one for each organ of my body. They were like visiting school inspectors, their residents and interns trailing close by. They studied my chart judiciously. They pored through my notes every day. I would watch them through my ICU glass window. After they were done with my chart, they would enter my room, ask the same routine questions, then leave. I felt like a specimen under a microscope.

But then there she was, my nutritionist. It would seem like she held the least consequential job among all my doctors. She was pulled in last to be part of my team. She had an air of youth about her. I hardly saw her pore heavily into my notes, but she came in my dark, cold room, pulled up a chair and talked about the vendor who always passed by her house to sell bread. One day, she noticed he didn't pass by her house any more. Later, she heard he'd had a stroke. One day, while strolling along in the market, she saw the vendor ambling along, selling his delicacies. He could walk again. He had to, for the sake of his children.

She asked what I did and what I still wanted to do. I had not thought far enough into my shaky future to know what I wanted to do with my changed self. But she talked of my stroke in a different light. She talked of a phoenix rising from the ashes. She talked of a life suddenly picking up its momentum. No one had bothered to talk to me like that—as a human. She reminded me of my humanity. I cried, fully acknowledging my grief for the first time. It resided in knowing what I had lost. But in that very dark cave, she showed me what could be. She glowed. It was clear that she wore being a doctor differently.

10

I stayed in the ICU for about three weeks. I had an elaborate plan how I was going to take the resident who *mishandled* me down. I came to the ER around 9.30 p.m. and was taken for an MRI near morning, around 4.45 a.m., when the MRI room, I learned, was readily available. I planned to request the hospital for my file, which was becoming thicker as the days passed by. I planned to look at the time I came in and the time I was attended to. If all the medical staff did was meticulously *endorse* me to the next person-in-charge, surely the times and dates I was handled would be duly recorded in my file. I planned to get her name. I planned who will handle my case. I asked my sisters to call my classmates up to make my case. I knew I was going to win. I even had a precedent for it, and I had taught it. I was going to enlist my best students to help me with the case. I pointed haphazardly to the letters in the communication board spelling, *I will sue her with a vengeance she doesn't know.* I was mad and determined. I wanted to make sure her career was lost forever.

My family tried to appease me and keep me positive by dissuading me against suing, but when all their efforts failed, my youngest sister, Mimi, would take my side. 'We will make sure she never practises again.' I knew of nothing else that reminded me of times before the stroke than suing.

11

I noticed my hearing getting cloudy. The sounds came a bit muted. I was worried that it was the beginning of another downward spiral. I was afraid I was becoming deaf. My hearing was the last good sense I had. I could not bear to lose it. I could barely see, but by my good hearing, I was relatively aware of everything. I asked to see my ear doctor. He had gone on vacation and sent his resident. The tools to have me checked were at the doctor's clinic which was then closed. The resident chalked up my reduced hearing to a clogged nose and some earwax. He prescribed some ordinary nasal spray. Some comfort it gave me that time, but gladly, the mild cloudiness did not progress to deafness.

12

I was adjusted to the daily grind. I knew all the nurses' names and their shifts, when it started and when it ended. Every time the nurses would inject something in me, they would always utter '*gamay*', warning me in Visayan that whatever they were jabbing at me would hurt a little. I loved all my nurses. I knew who loved BTS, who this male resident fancied, who loved to sing, who liked to trade stories while cleaning me. I knew them all. I started carrying slurred conversations with them. I didn't mind that my food and travel videos played repetitively on my TV screen. I began making travel plans for Christmas, naively thinking I could walk by then. Christmas, after all, was still a good three-quarters of the year away. I began fantasizing about coffee in the morning. I thought I had heard my nutritionist prescribe some for me through my NGT. Some interesting coffee drip it would have made. I was in maintenance. They were preserving the status quo. I was three weeks in since admission.

Meanwhile, Mimi contacted a doctor in a public hospital in Singapore to see if she would take my case. Since Singapore could only then accept their own citizens in public hospitals near the end of the pandemic, she referred me to a doctor in a private hospital. He held a remote meeting to check how I was. He agreed to take me in as his patient, but I had to be cleared by all my Philippine doctors to fly to Singapore.

Because all my tests were not telling my Philippine doctors what kept causing my strokes, they reached the conclusion that

I had vasculitis, a super rare disease that could provide the only explanation. I was too young and did not exhibit the risk factors for stroke. They thought my immune system attacked my healthy blood vessels, causing them to become swollen and narrow. To treat it, they wanted me on *Rituximab*, a drug that would plunge my immune system to basically nil but would lessen the swelling of my blood vessels. A nurse would have to monitor me closely as the medicine would drip to my veins. The drug would be on top of the maximum dose of steroids that I was already on.

To be able to take the medicine, they subjected me to numerous tests to ensure that I had no current infection. They sent my sputum to Manila. A test revealed that I had been harbouring bacteria in my chest from being exposed too long in the hospital. They treated it with antibiotics and waited for it to die before I was to start on *Rituximab*. They put a special air purifier in my room to keep me from infections of any kind. One day, my Philippine doctors reached a consensus just to give me the medicine despite the hospital-acquired pneumonia as long as I didn't have more threatening infections. I suppose they chose the lesser evil. But since we obtained all clearances to fly to Singapore that day, they decided to just have the drug administered when we got there.

I was hesitant to leave the nest. An entirely new culture at a new hospital at a new place. An entirely new ecosystem. I felt like I had to start from square one.

Part 2

13

There was excitement in the air, but I was not going for some travel or sabbatical. I was to be air-lifted by air ambulance to Singapore in a couple of hours. Before then, I had to be transferred to an ambulance to get me to the airport. The nurses hurried around to get me ready. They bagged my medicine, packed my milk, said their well-wishes and primed me to go. They issued me my discharge papers after approximately twenty-four hours.

The hour finally arrived, and an army medic and a blue-frocked doctor arrived to fetch me. The doctor was accompanying me on the trip. The nurses waved their goodbyes. It was a bittersweet farewell. No one wanted to overextend their visit, least of all me, but I didn't want to leave the comforts of the ICU as I had known it either.

If my whole life was a movie, this would be the moment worthy of the big screen, with the bustle of authorities around me. I was transferred from my bed to the stretcher and was wheeled out the door of the ICU. I was brought in through the back door of this dingy ambulance with faulty air conditioning, where I had to lay supine. We parked in a barren parking lot of this isolated airport. Literally strapped to the stretcher, I waited and waited, sick with the heat and the stale air inside the ambulance. The plane that was supposed to fetch me was delayed. My saliva started pooling at the back of my throat, and I still had four plus hours to Singapore on the plane.

Finally, the ambulance doors burst open and Turkish medics hurriedly came to me. 'How are you doing, Tracy?' I was surprised that someone had said my name outside of the hospital or said my name at all to me. It was exactly one of those scenes that you see in those medical shows—of a medic bursting in an ambulance's doors. As they pulled my stretcher out, I suddenly found myself facing the wide blue sky. I was being wheeled on the runway, feeling fresh air above me and beside me. It didn't matter that a couple of men scurried about me trying to get me into the plane. Nothing could budge me. The view was already infinitely better than anything in the hospital.

14

Up in the air, I decided to keep my small window open. It was just blue sky interspersed with white clouds, but it was captivating. My mom, sister, and two medics were with me on the plane. The medics served them cookies and chips. And me, my medicine served 36,000 feet above sea level. It was better than a commercial flight. We had the plane to ourselves.

Four hours on the plane and the same view. My main concern then was craning my neck to the left and to the right so it would not hurt. Except I couldn't look to the right for too long or else I would be staring at the scruffy medic. The plane was that small.

We landed in Singapore to be fetched by a new ambulance, two medics, and a sprightly young doctor. The medic was surprised that it was a young lady on a stretcher from her own country who had arrived. I guess she had expected some rich old mogul to land on their runway.

I breezed through immigration. Special perks of coming through an ambulance. I guess this was first world. What took hours back in my country took minutes in the private hospital that I was rushed in. I was whisked away to the ICU and underwent a series of random tests to ensure that I was clean and safe. The borders had just opened the previous week.

They swiped my anus with what felt like a long cotton bud. I found myself cold and alone in a new country. And this was just at the beginning.

15

I lay flat on my back as bright lights flashed before me. I was like a specimen in a Petri dish. *What was wrong with me?*

'We will get to the bottom of this before the night is over,' Dr Wee, the covering doctor, said. He was tall and lanky. 'The millennial doctor', they called him. He was methodical and scientific. *Did you get a neck massage before the stroke? Did you get into an accident before the stroke? What were your hobbies before the stroke?* He recounted the events from the episode of my stroke until he said, 'and it all went downhill from there.' I stopped in my tracks. *And it all went downhill from there?* He talked of a third stroke. I was still at the second. The first was undetected by the first MRI scan when I was rushed to the ER. The second was the larger stroke, large enough to be detected, which we welcomed ironically. I didn't know of a third. He said they had found a third stroke in the MRI scan that I brought from home. I was in the blind. The sad thing was I was conscious about the changes in my body as a result of my subsequent strokes and alerted the doctors about them as they were happening. I came to the hospital with just muscle weakness on my left but came out with practically all my four limbs immobile, barely seeing, speaking, eating, peeing, and pooing on my own. Out of all my experiences in the hospital, it is still the most bitter pill to swallow—bearing witness to how I lost function little by little in the best place I could be. It was like watching promise slowly seep down the drain.

Dr Wee ordered an MRI done on me, plus the changing of my catheter, oxygen cannula, NGT, and other appurtenances for new ones. It was hard enough the first time they were inserted, but I had to have it another time, alone and while unknown to the nurses. I was only a body to crowd in. The nurses were Chinese and Malay. They spoke in languages I didn't understand. I remember scraping my head for Mandarin learned in grade school to tell them what I needed.

Like an object in a factory line, they gave me a very quick wipe for a bath and removed my diaper. Four nurses crowded over my vagina, and after a quick discussion and a swiftness of hand, removed my old catheter and replaced it with a new one. People think that a body barely moving, with lips barely talking, cannot feel anything, but I felt every sleight of hand. I felt like nothing short of an animal, like a cow, pushed and shoved here and there. They were transactional. They were trying to save a function of me, but me, they couldn't care less about.

They took out my NGT in one nostril as they inserted the new one in the other nostril. I guess that's the price you pay for efficiency. It's not exactly the most compassionate route.

They needed to run some tests. A doctor came up to draw blood from me. They tried my arms. It was a sea of bruises of various colours. My veins were battered, but they needed the blood. Nonetheless, they took a chance on one. The needle pierced my skin, but my blood came in drops. The doctor tried to squeeze my arm desperately, as if encouraging my arm to produce the quantity he needed. 'She is so dry,' the thin Malay nurse said. It was eleven in the evening, and I had not been fed since before noon in anticipation of the air transfer. The medics had chosen not to give me my milk because they would rather I not feel nauseous up in the air. When they couldn't get the required quantity of blood from my veins, the doctor drew the needle through my femur, and I gasped at the pain.

It was past 1 a.m. when I was done with all my tests. They put a tissue box at arm's reach for my secretions, a plastic bag for a makeshift waste bin at the side of my bed, but I could barely raise my left arm, let alone carry a tissue. *How was I supposed to get through the night?* The nurses left me alone in my room for the rest of the night. Before they left, they switched on the television to the only English-speaking channel. It had on a gory mafia movie, where everybody got killed in the end. I wanted to switch the channel or turn off the television, but I had neither the control nor the strength to press the buttons on the remote, and I was too weak to press the button to summon the nurse. So, I finished the entire movie and did not get a wink of sleep on my first night before the morning nurse drew the curtain.

16

A bustle of activity jolted me back to my senses. It was the nurses' morning turnover. It was morning. The morning nurse was Filipino. It was a comfort to hear her. She was like a piece of home in a foreign land. She was thoroughly alarmed that I was young and yet had experienced a stroke. She had just survived cancer and saw illness for what it was. She was extra comforting, always did the extra mile when no one expected her to. She was my mom in that ICU.

Dr Wee came in at exactly 9 a.m. He had the results of the MRI from the night before. I had an arterial dissection; the lining of an artery in my neck tore. Blood clots formed at the site of the tear, travelled to my brain, and blocked off its supply of oxygen and nutrients, causing an ischemic stroke. I was to be under observation in the ICU for one more night.

I looked at the clock. A little past nine-thirty. Visiting hours were not until twelve noon, and it lasted only until 2 p.m. I never felt time move slower. I would stare away from the clock, whiling away what I thought was considerable time, only to return to it seeing only a few minutes had passed. No matter how I stared at the digital, neon numbers indicating the time, I could not will it to move faster. I was alone with nothing to do for the time being. I was stuck to my bed, invalid, expected to while away the time, just like that. I remember when I could still move, I would remark, *Where did the time go?* How funny that time was so accurate and yet so relative.

The opaque curtains drew open. Visiting hours were open, and my mom and sister bolted in with every intention to make use of the minutes. The moment the curtains closed, I broke into a sob. All my pent-up feelings finally broke loose after a harrowing night, being violated in every sense, and yet expected to hold it together like a corpse. Having a stroke is like staring death in the face and surviving what's left of you. You bear the traces of death, and yet you are still alive. Your family around you can't grieve and be left alone because there is still your derelict body to reckon with.

I could not hold it together. It was a pain incompressible in words. It was the cry of a child who lost her mother in a crowded marketplace. I had never felt so alone. The night when they replaced my catheter and NGT, I chanted to myself a line in a children's storybook that a friend had sent to me while in the ICU. *You only need to be tough for a little while.* I did not feel the need to summon my inner strength when I gagged from suction tubes that went too deep, when phlegm seemed to lodge in a cavity in my chest, but I needed to summon it that first night. I had no one to gather strength from but myself. I needed to be there for myself.

My mom desperately tried to extend her visit. She pretended that she was still waiting for my doctor if only to be allowed longer in the ICU. The guards in the hospital were relentless. They roamed the place like hawks to signal the end of visiting hours. A lady guard marked my mother as a recidivist. No sooner would the guard let my mom out, she would find her way back in again. They were like a cat and a mouse playing their game. The guard knew she had a job to do, but she was probably a mother too and knew all too well what my mother was feeling. 'My heart breaks,' was all she could muster as she gently let my mother out.

During that visit, knowing I would be alone for the second time, my mom and sister prepared me for the night to come. They wrote on Post-it signs stating 'Play Me' with reference to a USB filled with Christian services and Sandy Daza's[2] *Foodprints* and *Casa Daza* food videos for me to watch that night. It was for the nurse to find when I couldn't open my lips to speak what I wanted. It was a young Filipino nurse who was in charge of me that night. She put on the USB, and I listened ardently to the Christian service that night. It was calming and soothing, like a lullaby. It made me feel safe, and in a few minutes, I was sound asleep.

The nurses had prepared a cowbell for me that made it easier for me to press the call button to call them. Since the cowbell was not attached to their internal system, I had to ring the cowbell when a nurse was incidentally passing by. They put on me what seemed like bubble shoes and brushed my teeth with anti-septic cotton buds twice a day. I had never felt so taken care of, yet forsaken, in my whole life.

That second night, all I did was sleep. I asked if I could sleep through my bath. All the adrenaline from the previous night seemed to have drained from me. I woke in the middle of the night because I felt a tightness in my chest. I could not identify whether I was having a heart attack or some other disease. Later, I would learn that a brainstem stroke affected breathing. I had forgotten how to breathe normally, the presupposition of all life. The night nurse tried to allay my fears by talking me through my episode, until my heart rate lowered and my breathing evened out. She asked me how I became sick and told me how she had the same auto-immune disease as me. I knew what she was doing, but was grateful, nonetheless. I had her company.

I could never figure out if the tingles in my left arm were worsening or increasing. One time, I felt like the tingles

---

[2] My family met the chef—to my utter delight—in Singapore. I was obsessed with him in the ICU. He was billeted in the same hotel as my family. My nurse remarked that the first time that I slept really well in the hospital was when he sent a video greeting me. I wrote to thank him: 'In good times and in bad, your food uplifts.'

were increasing in my hand, and the nurse alerted Dr Wee, who immediately came to see me, fearing that my stroke had taken a turn for the worse. He checked my fingers. The tingles felt like electricity running through my fingers. Anything I touched felt charged to me. I thus did not know whether a part of my body tingled at touching something or if it tingled anew by itself. I was constantly scared that the tingles were spreading further and causing progressing immobility. 'It waxes and wanes,' explained Dr Wee.

An immunologist, Dr Lui, was pulled in to test if I had vasculitis. He ordered blood tests and a PET scan. The PET scan would show if my blood vessels were indeed swollen. A radioactive drug or a tracer was injected in a vein in my hand. The nurse tried several times to insert an IV line into my hand. First the left hand, then the right. My veins were so bruised and battered that they were loath to accept another foreign article into my body. My mother petted me to comfort me, but I felt only her anxiety and fear in her hands. In my stoic state, I assumed I was more a comfort to her during those times. We waited for about an hour until the tracer ran through my whole body. Then I entered this intimidating, giant, white, cold contraption. It was as harmless as an MRI, but it was like an oracle. It knew too much. The results came out. *I had no vasculitis. I did not need to take Rituximab.*

17

Arrangements were made for me to move to the general neurology ward. The nurses there were supposed to be experts on neurological diseases and knew how to handle neurological patients. Two of my nurses brought me down to the eighth floor—Zenaida and Jess. Two nurses that were hard for me to part with, because in two days, they had become family. I felt safe and known with them. 'How romantic,' the new nurse said sarcastically as Zenaida and Jess held my hands and said their goodbyes. 'Your life isn't over,' Zenaida whispered.

The nurses at the new ward were curt and impersonal. I felt as though a new task had just begun. I had to get to know them one by one and make them comfortable around me. A piece of my old self I carried with me. I felt like the host of my 24/7 party.

It turns out I had to shed my embarrassment several times before I was free. I turned on the television every time a new nurse opened my diaper and cleaned me. I don't know who the television was for, the nurse or for me. I shed my embarrassment layer by layer, until only the kernel of my existence remained. I was ready to be a child again. Like a baby, who does not know what to be ashamed of, I was shorn of all shame.

First things first. I needed to be off my catheter. The bladder muscles were intimately tied to the rectal muscles so they had to make sure all my poo was out before my pee could come out. So, they put me on oral medicine to induce me to poop. It was incredibly uncomfortable not knowing when it would come out.

I was doing occupational therapy, my legs being stretched here and there on the bed, when a pungent smell wafted in the air. 'I think she passed motion,' the therapist said matter-of-factly. There was no holding it. Pride, or any form of it, simply had to go.

The oral medicine wasn't enough. They put me on a suppository. My last recollection of being inserted with one was when I was five years old. I never expected that I would have to relive the discomfort when I was grown. Dr Wee came, and I told him I pooped twice. He sympathetically told me, 'I am afraid that's not enough.' He ordered that I be given an enema. I eyed the bottle suspiciously as it was about to be given to me. The enema was in a bullet-tipped bottle, which the nurse then injected in my butthole. The liquid the bottle spurted was supposed to meld with whatever remained in my intestines and, in twenty minutes, wash them away. Mine didn't take that long though. Immediately, a cramp spread through my abdomen, and I held the bars beside my hospital bed with white-washed knuckles, as I writhed and crumpled in pain.

The doctor got what he wanted. I was now expected to pee on my own. I had a window of six hours to pee. We listened to pee-inducing videos on YouTube but to no avail. We turned on the faucet to induce urination. Nothing. The nurses checked my bladder. Good thing it was not yet distended.

To make things more complicated, I had my menstruation when they wanted my pee from me. The blood apparently came out from another hole, and I didn't know whether the droplets coming out of me was blood or urine. I couldn't distinguish. All I knew was that it burned. I felt like an orange being squeezed out of its juice. The pain was intermittent; it would come every time the blood came out. The blood felt acidic, and I felt a distinct discomfort in my butt the whole time.

The doctor came and peeked into my butt hole and said matter-of-factly that there was stool coming out, and that must be where the discomfort was coming from. Moreover, I found I had urinary tract infection, which caused the burning sensation every time I peed. My right leg would bolt straight at the pain. I would brace myself for every pain expected.

I didn't have the liberty to change diapers each time. A putrid smell, sharp and chemical, would accompany me while doing physiotherapy. I had to act dignified as my therapist kneeled over to support my knee. I was embarrassed to say the least, but there were different standards of embarrassment now for us.

My pee and poo were like gold to the nurses. They tracked it as if their lives depended on it. If I didn't poo twice a day, they would give me the suppository they jokingly called the bullet. Sometimes they would wake me at dawn, urging me to pee by tapping my bladder so they could write something on their report before they checked out for the day. Some days they would need a urine sample from me. I had to give it to them clean and its integrity unquestioned, so I had to give it horizontally with my legs wide open as a nurse waited for my urine to spurt out to a plastic container. If it didn't come out that way, I had to give it while standing up, as a nurse waited below with a cardboard contraption to catch my liquid gold. I felt like nothing short of a goat.

My right limbs were as immobile as stone. I lost all control of them, but they were perpetually attached to my body. My arm would flail in all directions as I struggled to get up. Knowing I could not rely on it, I would forget it like a useless branch, prompting my nurses to bellow, 'Your arm! Your arm!' I had to rely on my left for a lot of things. My left knee suddenly carried double its load. I felt my muscles tear and build stronger ones. As I got up from the bed, I put all my weight on my left knee because I could not even control my right ankle to stay flat on the floor. It would twist and turn every chance it got.

The right side of my face could not feel temperature as the left did. My doctor put a cold can of Coke on my left and right cheek to check if it felt the same temperature to me. It was icy cold on my left but barely cold on my right cheek. My right foot was cold and swollen, as if some forgotten part of my body was in a biting freezer. I was immune to the cold. I would tear off my blanket with nothing but the thin cloth of my hospital gown to shield me from it. My family would bundle up with their hoodies and their blankets to survive in the freezing temperature I thrived in.

That's the deal with God's wrath. I've got to go through the suffering myself. Everyone can play the supporting character, but I've got to play the main role. We talk of the cross, but we talk less of enduring the cross. Such is the nature of suffering. I can't dip my head in the water and momentarily surface for air. Suffering is being immersed in mire and not knowing if I can get up.

18

The morning after I was moved to the neurology ward, a bulky senior nurse trudged in my room and drew open the curtains. Light streamed in my room. 'Do you want to take a shower?' she asked. Of course, I jumped at the chance at a shower. Bedridden residents only got to be showered once a week.

She held me by the hand and helped me to get up. *Oh, she meant an actual shower.* I thought she was going to give me a hair bath like the ones you get in the salon. I laughed to myself. I could barely sit up, let alone stand, and she was asking me to cross the room to shower. She was actually annoyed that I was not up and ready to go by 7 a.m. It meant I couldn't finish all my rehabilitation activities for the day. In the Philippines, I was still in my bed at 9 a.m., and the earliest doctor came then.

It became a family anecdote, that story. I guess that's how they did it in the first world. You can't be lackadaisical when you're actually trying to save lives.

19

Every morning at 5.30 a.m., a night nurse would noisily break into the dark of my room to wash me. I could opt not to take a shower, but I had to be all ready when the day nurses came at 7 a.m. By 7.45 a.m., my occupational therapist, Edward, would knock on my door ready for the day's session. He was a kind man, thin and lanky. He taught me everything I needed to know in that hospital. He was like a balm for me. He exuded a calming force. He put some semblance of order in my now disordered life.

The big event for the day for me now was physiotherapy. My physiotherapist was this sprightly, noisy character, who demanded what then felt impossible for me. I would wait for hours for physiotherapy, idly watching television, but also being painfully aware of the time.

I remember the first time I was allowed to sit for two hours at a time. It was the first time I saw the view out my window. I could finally make out the roads that my family traversed to the hospital daily. I could finally see the bottoms of the tall buildings that competed for space in my window. We adjusted my wheelchair so I could watch Netflix comfortably. I was watching a pizza show, with celebrities teaching me how to make one. I don't remember much of the show. Just that I was happy I could carry my back and my head for two hours at a time. It was like juggling a book atop my head, except the book this time was my head, and I was strengthening the wires in my neck to carry it.

My disability was a reckoning of sorts that revealed itself to me in stages. My physiotherapist would ask me to perform a certain movement, and after an awkward pause, I would find that I couldn't do it. My brain had stopped communicating with my limbs. No matter how much I tried, my brain signals couldn't reach my toes. The connection was lost. I was effectively a scarecrow, without a functioning brain centre.

The physiotherapist at the hospital pushed me to my limits. My dominant side was affected so I had to learn and rely on my left for everything. One session was particularly intense. My left, which was suffering weakness on its own, was struggling to carry the weight of my right. It had no strength yet to do the vigorous exercises asked of me. My left knee trembled at the enormous pressure it was in. It was all coming at me too fast.

The physiotherapy session ended with me persevering until the end, but the moment I returned to my room and the door closed behind me, I sobbed like a baby. I felt entitled in feeling threatened and unreasonable. I felt like I was losing my last good knee, the one I depended on for everything. It was throbbing and wobbling. I could not afford to lose it. Just when my sob broke, the door opened, and there was the physiotherapist I was crying about. She had come to see if I was okay. Apparently, someone had tipped her off to the fact that I was not doing okay, and she wanted to speak to me. Then and there I felt the last strands of my privacy dematerialize before me. In my most private and unguarded moment, I was there for all the world to see. I instantly composed myself, acting like how an acceptable person in the adult world would act. I felt resigned to my fate.

The next day, as I wrote my name with my left hand, covering the entire half of the newspaper, I stared at my handwriting and tears started rolling down my cheeks. It came from a sadness so deep, each tear was drawn from a well of it.

The most mundane things became gargantuan to me. 'Ring the nurse for everything.' The nurses would bear the brunt if a patient fell to the ground. I couldn't get up by myself. Edward helped me prop myself up from my bed and swiftly transfer my dead weight to my wheelchair. At night, I slept at a thirty-degree angle to ensure any saliva just flowed out the side of my mouth and didn't go to my lungs. My mom would be ready with a tissue for me to spit on after every couple of seconds. I would be awoken in between naps because of my own saliva. If I ever felt pity for myself, it was at this time.

20

Speech therapy was always a therapy I welcomed. My speech therapist, Hui Yong, was a tall, thin lady with short, flappy hair, who became my confidante in the hospital. She was the outsider who bore the brunt of what little news originated in the confines of my room.

Hui Yong's most immediate goal then was to make me swallow. I was still on NGT then, which I wore everywhere like a nose piercing. As I tried to swallow, I stared at the greeting cards my friends had written me, which Kim had posted on the wall before me. I don't know what I was trying to draw from the wall. Maybe my loved ones' sentiments held a special power, begging the universe to heal me. Whatever it was, I figured there must be some strength in people still wanting me to live. I stared hard at the wall during every attempted swallow. I imagined swallowing an entire fish ball or golf ball. I waited to feel a click in my throat.

I did musical scales as Hui Yong advised. My mom was relentless, urging me to do them fifty times instead of the ten that had been advised. I did chin tucks with a plastic lever. She put nodes and ran electricity over my throat.

I sang karaoke. I felt like a frog croaking. Each syllable carried several pitches and contained an innate vibrato. I chased and gasped after the words. I could barely let out the first word when the next line started.

Later, a nurse would confess that she was afraid for the girl down the hall who could not even swallow her own saliva.

Hui Yong would tell me months later that she was terrified for me, when she had first met me in the ICU. I had been confined for about one month in the hospital back in Cebu and still didn't have a trace of the ability to swallow. But of course, she didn't tell me what she thought then. She kept it to herself. You don't say that to someone who's still trying, who places the remainder of themselves on the line to get a semblance of what was. Hope is a delicate thing.

21

It was interesting to be in the neurology ward. How many curious cases the nurses must see every day. I remember laying immobile in my bed, just before falling sleep, and hearing groans of anguish or pain from my next-door neighbour. The walls were thick, but not thick enough to conceal his devastation. I wonder if you are beset by some neurological disease, whether you can still characterize your pain as devastating. I should think it more merciful if the pain stays in some biological, physiological realm. I could pity myself, but I seemed to be well within our ward's standards.

On the way to rehab, this man handcuffed by the railing in front of the nurses' ward piqued my interest. He seemed totally respectable, with wire-rimmed spectacles, reading the day's paper as if in his office. I wondered how he handled the stares from people who passed by him in the halls. Apparently, the nurses handcuffed him to keep him in their sight always. He was prone to do a lot of dangerous (or indecent) things when left alone in his room. The night before he was rumoured to have walked the halls naked, frightening everyone. His wife had to go to work, so he was alone most of the day. You would think he was beset by some rare, grave neurological illness, but, in fact, he just lacked an essential electrolyte in the body—potassium. Once he was infused with it, he returned to a completely normal state.

22

For the life of me, I didn't know how diapers worked. I didn't know how to poop without space for the poop to fall into. I just couldn't wrap my head around it logically. I certainly did not want to bathe in my own poop. I kept on leaning to the side, giving space for my poop to spring out. I used to dread feeling the urge while seated. It was like summoning all your strength only to find yourself rooted to a chair. It's not like I had much choice. It was either on the chair or on the bed, and good luck figuring out how to do it horizontally.

I would go around the hospital and learn that the faucet had to leak. I would return to my room with my diaper, hospital gown, and the seat of my wheelchair soaked. My diaper couldn't contain all that I had to give. It took all my effort to get up on the bed to be changed then return to my wheelchair for the activities of the day. It was like being on a marathon but not of my own volition.

My diaper days were soon to meet their sunset days, however. Transitioning from diaper to no diaper took time and effort. Edward guided me. I was to pee before his session started whether I felt the urge or not. I was to seat myself at the toilet the same time each day whether I felt the urge to go or not. In between, I had to manage. I could barely trudge through the short distance from the dresser where I'd be seated to my washroom. Every time I would feel an urge, we would make a mad dash. If Kim adjusted my foot a second too long in the toilet, my urge would be gone. I had to ring the nurse each time I wanted to go. The nurse would keep the door open but attempt to give me some privacy by drawing a thin curtain on the door. But some privacy it was. I would catch her blatantly keeping a watchful eye on me through a slit in the curtain.

One day, I felt the urge. I begged Kim not to call the nurse so we could make it to the bathroom on our own, and I could have a little privacy while defecating. Maybe that way I'd actually be successful. But she couldn't risk my falling to the floor, so it had to be a team effort with the nurses. A nurse transferred me haphazardly to the commode with wheels to bring me to the toilet in time. Well, we all tried. You've got to reward effort. My poop leaked out, leaving my poor sister to scoop my sordid mess from the floor. How many people do you think you could count who have done that in their lifetimes? It looked exactly like the emoji, she mused, some swirling mountain of poop. I can now be embarrassed by almost nothing.

23

I joked that I had never been busier than I was in the hospital. The nurses had to chase me at the gym to give me my milk, medication, or to draw my blood. One time, I was strapped to a robot helping me to walk when a nurse came in complete with what seemed like his portable nurses' station. He then struck a needle to an exposed area of my arm and drew blood as I sat there. It looked like Ironman needing to go to the nurses' office. It was par for the course. In real life, being strapped in an Ironman suit with a nurse drawing blood nearby—you don't exactly see this in the streets. It was a different reality in the hospital, but an all-too-real reality just the same.

When I was finished with all the therapies and medical procedures for the day, I'd switch off, and immediately this free-as-a-bird feeling would swell over me, like a schoolgirl having the afternoon off. Now, there were only a few places to go take off in the hospital. There was the fruit shop run by two elderly ladies. Suffice to state, it was like Charlie's chocolate factory for those of us who were not so lucky.

Then there was the tiny French bakery that didn't have most of what was on its menu, but its aroma on the way to the hospital garden was just so enticing that I had to stop before its glass windows that were filled with glossy pastries, even if they were the same pastries every day. I must have been a sight to behold for the other customers. This girl with a tube down her nose staring at the glass windows, longing for what she could not have. But longing, back then, was enough for me. The smells of the bakery filled me. It felt as if the cool citrus cream sat on my tastebuds. I could pass by the bakery just to get a sniff of that warm, bitter coffee aroma lingering in the air. I loved watching busy doctors getting their fix as they hastily started their busy lives; distressed families taking a brief respite from their tough realities. I used to be one of them, until I became a patient.

I always made sure to pick a pastry, even if I could not eat it. My family always obliged my tastes. The bakery was on the way to a tiny garden with a bridge straddling a tiny man-made pond. Well, it was more pavement than garden really, but it was the highlight of my day. Often times, Kim would share a Danish and a coffee there with me. People would come and go from the garden—normal people presumably visiting their sick loved ones, munching quietly on their pastry, alone with their thoughts; patients like me in their hospital robes, just feeling the sun on their skin before they headed back to their air-conditioned rooms; sombre family members hoping to catch a glimmer of hope from thin air; transients at the hospital, just taking a test or two. Whoever there was in the garden that day, they were something to me. I no longer had the normalcy to simply pass them by.

I would read aloud from the newspaper in the garden, letting the humid afternoon air receive my breathless sentences. I gasped for air after every two syllables. Sometimes I would take a marker with me and try to scribble my name on that day's paper. There was a tranquil communion between my soul and my God in those quiet, sunny sessions.

We were in a state-of-the-art hospital, but there really was nothing to do in that massive playground. With not many choices, we found ourselves at the end of the hall where three vending machines were. There was a boring coffee vending machine that was cheap and dependable. There was this OJ machine that squeezed fresh oranges when you ordered a drink. Then, there was this shining, bright-lit salad bar of a vending machine that dished out a variety of cold cut sandwiches, tuna pitas, chicken salads, and yogurts. It's amazing how little you need to make you happy.

When really pressed to the wall for leisurely activities, Kim would wheel me to the first floor where the parking spaces were visible from the tall glass walls in the lobby. We would take note of which doctor drove which kind of luxury car.

I will always think fondly of that place. The stinging antiseptic smell of the hospital will always welcome me. It was my ecosystem for the longest time, a maze I could get lost in safely, a place I could aptly call home.

24

My faith was shown to me. No one could go through what I went through without having a crisis of faith. I was thrust in a situation, where, in an abyss, I could choose to see or not to see God. In the ICU back home, I used service videos, which my family downloaded for me, to fall asleep. I would fall asleep as the first hums of the video played. The sermons no longer carried any credibility for me. Pain had now baptized me in a way it did not normal mortals. I could not string two sentences of prayer together, even if just in supplication. I did not look to Him for healing. I did not endow Him with that power. I was never as secular.

One day, Halina, a nurse whom I had grown chummy with, came in and brought a prayer card which she stuck at the rails beside my bed. That way, if my head just hung to the side, my eyes would land on it. 'Be beside me; be behind me; be in front of me', the prayer card read. It spoke to me in a way that felt so literal to me, as I was then learning to walk with people surrounding me at all sides. I felt my mind lighten up. My mother then asked me to say a prayer out loud before they left. *Help me, Lord, so I can swallow. Help me, Lord, so I can walk. Help me, Lord, so I can talk clearly. Help me, Lord, so I can see clearly. Help me, Lord, so I can pee. Help me, Lord, so I can poo.* Never had I prayed like that before the stroke. I needed Him for the most basic things. I cried hearing how deep in the pits I had fallen to. It was a few minutes where I understood how much of children we really are.

25

My Aunt Jan and Uncle Ed came to visit me one weekend in Singapore from San Francisco, having heard of my condition. Both were doctors and were extremely worried about me. As their weekend drew to a close, I bid them a good flight and goodbye. I tried to act casually up to the last minute, but I couldn't hold it in the end. Everything now was far from normal. They had known me as this bubbly character since I was a kid. They had to say goodbye to all that history and come to terms with this person in front of them, a trace of a vibrant past. I let loose the elephant in the room. I wailed, my pent-up emotions uncontrollable. As I burst into tears, a nurse came in and stayed in my room at that very intimate moment. Though she was quiet and meant to be respectful, I felt naked sharing that very private moment with her.

26

There was once a nurse who got transferred to our ward. I knew everybody, but she was a fresh face. I was used to everybody barging in and out of my door time and again; it no longer rattled me. But then a sound I hadn't heard for a long time reverberated in my room. I couldn't quite place the sound. It was familiar yet distant. I had never made much of a door knock before, but here it was, beautiful and halting before me. Yes, apparently, you could still have those sacred moments in the hospital.

27

I never felt fear like I felt in the hospital. I did not know my body. I could not trust my brain. I didn't know whether a feeling was a progression of my illness, something to cause alarm, or just something I should disregard and not bother people about. But the cost of second guessing and speaking too late were too great. I had spoken in time, and yet here I was with my four almost sedentary limbs. Only a select few know the feeling of having one's face droop before one's eyes, and not be able to do anything about it.

I thought I had chest pain, which plagued me more during the night than during the day. The doctor and nurses acted quickly. They performed an ECG and prepared to do a blood test on me. A young nurse tried to draw blood from me, and when she couldn't, a more senior nurse took over the syringe, and when duty called her elsewhere, a male nurse took over. I felt like a pit stop. Thankfully, nothing alarming could be found in the results, and my kind immunologist ordered a medicated patch to be plastered on my chest, if only to psychologically alleviate my fears.

Other days, I would wake up to a lingering headache which would cause the nurses to call the doctor in the middle of the night. I didn't know headaches any more. My stroke, after all, started with a subtle one, a minor discomfort that made me swivel on my pillow the night before. I didn't know if it was my position. I was contorted to different positions every two hours to avoid bed sores. I found myself making justifications for what I felt.

One night, I couldn't sleep because I thought I was having a headache. The nurse gave me my paracetamol. Immediately, I felt my chest heave. I thought I was having a heart attack. I looked at Kim, sleeping and exhausted on the hospital couch. I forced myself to focus on my breathing until, thankfully, I drifted off to a deep sleep.

I asked my doctor how I was to know that I was having another stroke instead of a harmless headache. He answered, 'If the headache is lingering, and it's something that a dose of Panadol can't fix, then you have something to worry about.' On the occasions I'd have a headache, I'd pop two tablets of Panadol. A wave of sleepiness would wash over me, but I would keep myself awake to make sure the pain would go away. I waited to make sure the paracetamol was not just a stop-gap measure.

Whenever I would close my eyes to sleep, my insides would start caving. Later, I would find that the moment my stomach started caving was the moment I started drifting off to sleep. But I didn't recognize that feeling then. It was all too original a sensation. Too many years we've been together, but I was being introduced to my body anew. I was literally born again.

28

Dr Lee, my primary doctor and neurologist, was my last connection to the outside world. He brought news from the outside and came to visit every day. Our day started early because Dr Lee came early. He came around 7.30 a.m. every day, which was early for us, considering the sun rose at 7 a.m. in Singapore.

Dr Lee was unlike any doctor I had met. He seemed to have time. If he was busy, he didn't let us know about it. In his brusque way, he would barge into our room and then linger. He would regale us with stories about his kids, his wife, his parents, his house. He talked of the soft-serve ice cream in the mall across, and how you had to get it from this particular lady to get it extra tall. He spoke often about the *saba* at the food court across and when best to line up for it. I had no idea how the mall across looked, nor had I any ambition to stride across to it any time soon, but he kept it in my reverie—assuring me that the landscape hadn't changed. He just kept it on pause for me.

'Go straight and left until the end,' he advised. 'Don't get distracted,' he told us with specificity where the saba stall was. He kept the conversation bubbly and jumping, that you just had to get to the stall. We hardly talked of the stroke. We kept an unspoken five-minute rule. We only talked about the stroke for the first five minutes and kept the rest of the time casual.

Yet, he wasn't an unfocused doctor. When I had a series of headaches, he ordered an MRI to be done on me. In the middle of the day, he came to my room to discuss the results line by line, all five paragraphs of them. It was clear to me that he took being a doctor to heart. Not for status. Not for money. But why doctors became doctors in the first place.

Knowing I loved to read, he dropped by the neurology gym one morning and brandished a neurological essay on ice cream. He read me a line that he had noted in advance. 'It is also true that in 1997 the British Medical Journal noted that "ice cream headaches" can be produced by cold temperatures on the back of the palate, which stimulate the sphenopalatine ganglion to dilate blood vessels in the brain. However, the article concluded with the heartening sentence "Ice cream abstinence is not indicated".'[3] I loved that essay. I practised reading it line by line in the garden, the sentences truncated by my short breaths. I tried to read it when my eyes still skipped every other line, such that I always had to go back to the line before to finish the essay. Suffice to say, he kept things light, like I still had a right to enjoy an essay on ice cream and not constantly stare back at the bombshell staring me in the face.

Whatever Dr Lee told me, whether consequential or silly, was news for the day. I would repeat it to my parents word for word when they arrived in my hospital room. It was also all I could talk about at speech therapy to Hui Yong. He gave me fodder to talk about in the hospital, anything to take my mind off myself and the extremely difficult situation I was in. He was not a grim figure bearing unpalatable news. Rather, he was what hospital visits were made of. I never knew you could look forward to a doctor's visits.

'Draw on your reserves,' he would advise. I would playfully counter, 'Where are they?' not knowing how in the world I was to activate something I did not know existed. It was like having a back-up server, but not knowing you had one. But he seemed sure. I had to trust him. He kept me floating every day in the meantime;

---

[3] Excerpted from Fadiman, A. (2008). *At Large and At Small: Familiar Essays*. Farrar, Straus and Giroux.

until I could locate my back-up server. He never looked back, never asked me what could have possibly caused the stroke. There could be a myriad of reasons, but none worth returning to. He kept me going forward.

29

I wish I could tell you it was all smooth sailing for me, but my ordeal was dotted with extreme hardships that not only made me question, but reject my faith.

I could not swallow. Peeing and pooing were insufferable. Normal people hardly thought of these things, yet it took all of me. I clung to the hospital bed rails and shook them angrily, not knowing how to get out of the desperate situation I was in. *If you are real, God, show yourself.* I had never felt more forsaken. Everyone empathized with me, but that was all that they could do. I was massively alone. No one else could get through it but me.

It would take my mom hours to calm me down after a tantrum. It was a pointless thing. After my bout of rage, I could only lie in my hospital bed tired, shattered, embarrassed, and dejected. They called it a release, but a release from what exactly, I did not know. Maybe the loss in my body had to be mourned, and that was the only way how. I had been at the cusp of life when it was so rudely snatched from me. Here I was, a young woman stuck to her wheelchair for the greater part of her life. You could not think of the life before me and not feel waste. My paralysed body kept me in a straitjacket, but come to think of it, I had been in a straitjacket long before that.

30

I had been on my NGT for a month now. Dr Lee and Hui Yong, had been warming me to the idea of getting a percutaneous endoscopic gastrostomy tube (PEG). It supposedly was a mild and easy operation that made feeding me easier. No need to pour milk through a tube in my nose and amuse the nurse while the milk drained down my nostrils for a solid twenty minutes. Feeding through a tube was an eating experience that was far from pleasurable. I hated the smell of vanilla milk, yet I had to endure feeding six times a day. A PEG would make eating less troublesome and a lot faster.

While Dr Lee and Hui Yong were juggling with the idea of a PEG, Hui Yong and I continued with our therapy sessions. I had not eaten in so long that I didn't crave anything, even if I smelled it. I did not long for the taste of home that Glenda, a nurse from home, always graciously shared with my family. There was the *puting adobo, paksiw, monggo,* and dried fish, with their strong smells permeating my room. They were mouth-watering dishes, but my tastebuds had practically died. Ironically, I kept watching foodie videos,[4] probably unconsciously thinking it would hasten my swallowing somehow.

Three weeks in, and not a single swallow. Hui Yong was as committed as she could be. She came even on her days off, just so I would not get waylaid in my progress. She talked to the nurse about not feeding me before her sessions, so that out of hunger,

---

[4] *Somebody Feed Phil* kept my tummy growling and my feet moving (figuratively).

I could swallow. Halina, who had been feeding me milk for a while now, studied me closely and quietly. 'Give her a chance,' she said.

I didn't know how I could have merited a chance, but I guess that's how liberality works. I was not used to how it works yet. I was used to meritocracy. I got what I deserved. But that time somebody else put her foot down for me. She was quite an influential veteran nurse, and she swayed Hui Yong to take her side. No PEG. 'Let's give her one more week,' she insisted. She turned off the television and made me concentrate.

So, we began with ice chips and my own saliva to swallow. I don't recall when the first tick happened, when my throat finally decided to open its floodgates, but I seemed to have hurdled it and found myself on the other side. Hui Yong sure was calm throughout the whole process, never wildly exciting me of my progress. She was very directed and collected. She asked me what I craved to eat. I gave it a serious thought. *Apples.* Out of all things, apples. She couldn't give me apples directly, but she could manage something close. She asked the hospital commissary for some apple slices, wrapped them in gauze, and asked me to suck the juice from them. Soon after, we tried ice cream, smooth so it could slide down the throat, then Coke and soda water, so that its bubbles would tickle me to swallow. Then, we graduated to bananas, thickened water, porridge with blended carrots, mashed potato with gravy, and later, a minced diet. I looked forward to hospital food like it was a gourmet meal I could finally eat.

I was swallowing. I couldn't believe it. I got a part of my life back. My tummy bloated, unused to the food. The first time I could eat a regular meal, I wolfed down everything they set before me—a banana, a yogurt, a main, a coffee, and a cheesecake. I pored heavily through the hospital menu and thought carefully about what I wanted to eat five times a day. I could even eat burgers, Hui Yong said.

Every swallow felt like a gift, but also a gamble. 'Doubly swallow,' Hui Yong advised if I wasn't sure I fully swallowed something. I constantly harassed Kim, asking if I had successfully swallowed my food. I didn't choke but there was always that feeling that something didn't go down the right tube. I was not used to how swallowing felt yet. As soon as I would burp, I would stop. It was a signal for me that my body could not take in more and that my muscles were less willing to participate in my feast.

I could eat so little, yet I felt my stomach walls hyper-extend. I struggled to do physiotherapy with so little sustaining me. I could not swallow water, so I only had sips of sugary drinks. The question now, was not whether or not I could swallow, but whether I could consume enough for my sustenance.

We set a soft date for my McDonalds party. When my NGT was to be removed, I somehow had fries in mind, as the first food from outside that was to grace my tummy. Hui Yong didn't renege on her promise. She over-delivered. We were about two weeks ahead of schedule for my NGT to be removed. A nurse came in to matter-of-factly remove my tube. She drew it out from me as if recovering something from the drainpipes from the sink at home. They were old and musty. It was time for them to see the light of day. There was no ceremony, but just like that, the faculty of taste was returned to me.

With the tube out, I struggled with swallowing liquids. There was no option. I had to swallow or else. My pills had to be cut so that I could swallow them easier. Each had to be put in a spoonful of yogurt or apple juice so it could just get flushed with the tide. I remembered my grandad who could swallow several pills at a time without water. Boy, was I a long way off but at least I had my foot in the door. I asked my parents to leave when it was time to swallow the pills. Their anxiety was too difficult for me to swallow.

One night, I decided to just have my pills in the bathroom while I was upright and seated in my commode. I swallowed all the hard ones and left the sticky, liquid one last. It tasted and had the consistency of corn syrup which I hated. I tried to drink it in one gulp when the sticky substance seemed to cover my air pipe. My eyes bulged, as if realizing what was happening to me and calling for help. I tried to breathe. Instead, I wheezed. Kim panicked, ran to the nurses' station, and called for help. The nurses ran to my aid. I coughed, hoping to bring up what was stuck in the wrong tube. In an attempt to appease the nurses, I forced a smile as if to say I was okay. I coughed some of the syrup, and they settled me in my hospital bed to calm me down, but I bolted right up knowing that something was still in the wrong tube. All through the night I coughed what was left of the syrup. *Was I aspirating?* Aspirating meant my lungs could get infected with a morsel of food or water. I would have to take strong antibiotics on the off chance it did not kill me. I stayed up past my bedtime that night watching soothing legal shows, holding fast to the life I held. In an instant it could be gone, and that night I was acutely made aware of that.

31

Times at the hospital weren't always depressing. I couldn't tell a lie to save myself. My leg would stiffen every time I was excited, angry, cold, or plain anxious. My flesh was like a transparent film. You could see through my heart. By God's grace, I guffawed a lot in the hospital. My therapist explained that you could either laugh or cry by the lack of inhibition. Good thing my burden was to stop laughing.

I laughed at everything. A face would tick me off, reminding me of a funny event, and it would ruin me. I hated being wheeled by my dad to the gym because he wheeled so slowly, taking his merciful time to say hi to everybody we passed, when I was in my wheelchair trying to hold it together. I would hold my breath behind my mask until my wheelchair would cross into the confines of my own room where I would burst into hysterical, boisterous laughter.

There was this kooky nurse, Kristine, who made the mistake of tickling my funny bone. I couldn't stop laughing just by seeing her. She had to stop herself from going into my room (I figured when I hardly saw her) because she obviously couldn't make herself useful while inside it. I would not stop laughing. Just seeing her in the corridors to the gym would trigger me. I would laugh all the way to the gym, passing by the nurses' station, with my head hung low, as if on the walk of shame. My laughs were accentuated with loud snorts that made my laugh utterly embarrassing. I reported to Dr Lee that I was laughing too much. *Could it be the Prozac?*

He assured me, though without any basis whatsoever, that it wasn't. I needed the Prozac to keep me motivated in my intensive rehabilitation to my great convenience.

I would burst into fits of laughter in the middle of therapy, prompting my therapist to pull a mirror in front of me to still me. I would focus on my reflection and try my hardest to appease myself and catch a semblance of that decent lady in me before the stroke. *Heck, I was a lawyer, for crying out loud*, I wanted to shout to myself. That image of me was slowly slipping away. I did not act my age. It would boggle my family watching me in rehab, laughing at whatever set me off in that silent, empty room. I would giggle in the middle of the night for no apparent reason. I would smile the moment I woke up and crack jokes from my hospital bed.

One time after finishing with my PET scan, the technicians forgot to put my denture and mask back on. I couldn't very well tell them that because I didn't want to remind them I was missing a tooth. My toothlessness was an inconvenient matter. It nestled in a very conspicuous place. I was missing a front tooth. I couldn't do much to keep myself looking legitimate because my face was half frozen. My appearance always jolted the technicians to a respectful state of suppressed laughter. Their eyes would crinkle while I tried to hold myself together because I didn't want to open my mouth and reveal my sting. Staff wheeled me back to my room. Like trained operatives, nurses from my ward received me. I motioned for Kim to at least put back my mask on, but she couldn't get a clue. My mother was just as hopeless. Obviously, I could not utter a word while serious business was happening in my room. I found it ludicrous that I was the stroke victim, and yet I was the only one with the presence of mind to remember my fake tooth. And then it happened. I could feel a giant fit overpowering my nerves. *How could I fight it?* It washed over me like a waterfall. I burst into laughter and gave up any hope of concealing my secret. The nurses all turned to look at me. I freely, and of my own volition, exposed myself.

I couldn't have been more grateful that my mind was on my side during my darkest times. I wonder how it would have been otherwise. It would have been easy to drown in the murk because the murk was dark and deep. I will have to thank my lack of inhibition someday, for choosing to be on the side of the light, when it was easier to stay in the shadow.

32

'It's not the walking that matters. Sure, can walk,' my physiotherapist clarified in her truncated English. 'It's the gait that matters.' And so, every day I studied how to walk, never knowing where my hip was, relative to my whole body. Normal people do not ever have to familiarize themselves with their joints, bones, and muscles in order to move them, but I did. Not knowing which muscle was for which action was hard enough but having to figure it out with my head half fried and with nothing moving made it infinitely harder. I spent my weekends learning to walk on my own when I didn't have therapy. 'No one works out seven days a week,' my physiotherapist mused. Not when you were in a roomful of desperate people. Rehab was a weeklong job. I traipsed around the small diameter of my room, passing by a small mirror in the dresser to survey my stance and posture.

One day, my physiotherapist took a leave of absence for feeling under the weather. Immediately, I felt my shoulders relax. I could learn how to walk without her barking over my ear. Only a young therapist and her assistant who I was chummy with were assigned for the day. With ease, I started walking to-and-fro across the gym with my covering therapist's hand clutching the back of my pants to prevent a fall. When we got to one end of the gym, I shuffled my feet to turn. I had trouble with walking but turning was my area of expertise. Somehow, it was easier to balance while turning.

And so, I turned, and somehow lost my footing. I felt myself tip over the edge like a log, cross over the point of no return. I could not disassociate my limbs. I felt myself lose balance. Because I had no means to save myself, because I could neither brace for nor prevent impact, I switched off. I blacked out. It was the last defence of my body. If it could not save itself, at least it could spare it the memory of the fall. The last thing I felt was my irretrievably falling and the petite therapist not having enough strength to pull me up. I felt her coming down with me.

The next thing I knew was myself being pulled up forcibly by the therapist assistant. My mom who had been at the other end of the gym ran to my end terrified. Therapists and therapist assistants crowded over me. My occasional speech therapist, Rae, who had grown to become a friend, offered me some water.

I would later learn that I had buried my head in my shoulders as a defence mechanism. It turns out I had something programmed within me to keep me from hurting myself. I didn't know it, but it sure knew to come out when needed. *Was it my reserve?* A therapist assistant, Yvonne, gave me chai latte to calm myself.

Since I was on blood thinners, the nurses checked my body constantly for bruising. I could have hit my head or suffered from internal bleeding from a slight bump. They erased their sign on their white board proudly stating that it had been 111 days since there was zero fall. The unlikeliest patient to fall, a young woman, had a fall. My neurologist was notified that I fell. Thankfully, my therapist and I came out unscathed from the accident.

That night I felt what faith means. It's like the mantle that protects you to make you invincible. I shudder to think of what could have happened to me, but I suffered not a single bruise. I could have hurt myself more easily at home. I looked back on my journey and saw that I had come a long way. At every point, never had I come out permanently scarred. I lost my sight but could now see. I lost my speech but could now talk. I lost bodily movement on the left but have since recovered it. My mind was intact despite the stroke. I had a recovery to look forward to despite being plunged in the deepest pits. For the first time, I felt, palpably, that nothing could hurt me. It was a feeling of safety and assuredness I had never felt before. A profound peace settled over me. I felt snug in His embrace.

33

I used to wonder why the feelings of shame came over me in the shower pre-stroke. It was not a feeling I carried with me all day, but when stripped to the core, there it was, bobbing its head. The feeling was unmistakable. It was like being born into society but not living up to the name. I was not concerned with my manner of dress enough. I didn't fancy social gatherings. I was not married. Time was running out, and I saw that prospects were slim, but I didn't want to be part of any of it.

When I came to be sick, the opposite dawned on me. Daily there were affirmations of who I was. My silliness and curiosity were my assets. My candidness drew people in with its authenticity. We got rid of the small talk and skipped right to the good stuff. I asked the tough embarrassing questions that one is not supposed to ask to preserve one's face in society. I made friendships I actually wanted to keep, friendships which I didn't need to take care of like a bunch of glass balls because the silence between us could take care of itself. I was sufficient. In fact, I was more than sufficient. I was thriving. This knowledge boosted my confidence in myself like no laurel ever did. It didn't feel earned. It was innate to me, this seed of potentiality waiting to be watered. It felt like stepping into the light when I was standing in the shadow all along. The light was always there, but I liked to skirt around it all this time. Perhaps the light was so bright that I didn't trust it, or I wanted others to step in with me. But the light was friendly and warm and solved all my problems bit by bit. It was time I stepped into my own inheritance.

34

One of the best things about having a stroke, mine at least, was having a blank brain. You could place a notebook in front of me, and I wouldn't have anything to write on it, except things you told me to. So I wrote inconsequential silly things in my notebook when I was having the most harrowing experience of my life.

I felt things, but I didn't grasp them. I knew things but didn't feel the gravity of them. My injured brain was like a balm masking my pain. I could only focus on the task at hand. So, when all activities subsided around 9 p.m. at night, when everybody had their fill of me, I asked Kim to turn off the lights, turn up the air conditioner, put on my blanket, wear her hoodie, and deliciously stream our favourite show on Netflix. That time, that show happened to be *Lincoln Lawyer*. It reminded me of how it felt to be a lawyer before. I had high cognitive skills for a stroke survivor, but I was dumb enough not to care about what was happening to me. I was chill enough to watch Netflix every night.

As I stayed longer in the hospital, my brain slowly understood the beating that I suffered. When somebody then described my situation as grave, it dawned on me that my situation was severe. It's funny how the brain doesn't know what blow it has taken until a label is put before it. *Moderate to severe stroke*. That's apparently what I had. I wrapped my head around it. Thank God I knew of it when I had endured the difficult part—the several MRIs where I had to steel myself not to move for more than an hour even though breathing was excessively difficult. In my toughest moments when I was under the MRI machine, I had called on the spirits of my two grandmothers to accompany me in my suffering. I had willed myself to stare at the tiny insect that somehow managed to intrude upon that cold, impersonal room and linger at the side of the white giant tube that swallowed me, if only to distract myself from the passing of time. I had endured my PET scan, after nurses scrambled to insert an IV in my battered veins. I had overcome a needle being poked in my finger before every meal and steroids being stabbed in my abdomen almost every day. I had graduated from the worst. I had survived it before feeling the punch of the blow.

I came to an unwavering faith that those suffering more than me must have a buffer to their suffering like an unknown covenant with God that no matter how bad it looked on the outside, one was still intact inside. He does not give us more than we can handle. I lived through that promise.

35

The day was ominous. They said someone was about to be discharged, and he was waiting for an auspicious day to go. The next day the government imposed a lockdown, and the poor guy ended up in the hospital for two more years before he left. My discharge was not as ceremonial. It was bittersweet. I had come to know all the nurses, therapists, and orderlies in the hospital. It was my new ecosystem, and I had grown to love them.

The day after I had fallen in the gym, a solicitous nurse advised, 'Just go. You shouldn't have given farewell pizza. Just quietly go.' People who are too loud in exiting suffer setbacks. I had given farewell lunches to the therapists and nurses the week before I left.

I wrote heartfelt letters to my doctors, nurses, and therapists. Since I couldn't write with my left, I ran what I wanted to say in my head and rehearsed them in my head until done. I asked Kim to write down my letters in empty cards. I had the chance to fill my brain anew, and they were the people who populated it. They rebuilt me. I wrote to Dr Lee:

Dear Dr Lee,

I hope you like flowers[5] because it is the only card that I have.

They say I have a fighting spirit, but I have none until I have nothing

---

[5] The card had an elaborate pop-up flower.

left to give. And then I know what Hebrews 11:1[6] truly means.

You are the best kind of doctor that I know. You gave me a diagnosis and your friendship.

I shall leave with three things with me:

(1) there are two kinds of people: tedious and charming;

(2) wake up at sunrise; go to bed at sun down;

(3) go to Takashimaya and buy Hokkaido ice cream. Someday, I'll buy you a cone.

I shall be grateful for you every year that I live. And lest you forget, you hold two rabbits under your hat because why not you?[7]

I shall miss your 'rubbish' every day.

Love,
Tracy

My last day went by like a breeze. All the nurses came out of their station to take a collective photo. They said their individual goodbyes, exchanged numbers, and took photos with me. My mom bumped into Dr Wee. He came up, and we took a photo with him making a fighting fist mid-air.

Dr Lui, my immunologist, came by the night before in his scrubs, when we had long turned off the lights, to say his goodbye. I told him I had no desire to return to the Philippines because of my harrowing time there. He kindly dismissed my comment and said, 'They did the best they could with the resources they have.' What he said was like cold water splashed on my face. He was sobering and empathetic at the same time. It's not about me all the time. My horrible circumstances were not a license for me to get a justified pass in life all the time.

---

[6] 'Now faith is confidence in what we hope for and assurance about what we do not see.', NIV.

[7] An inside joke.

I was already almost missing Dr Lee, who came by every day and inadvertently became my friend. I had been a test case for his students. I would dutifully act as the specimen for review, and when the whole scene was over, would ask him the next day, how the student fared. It was the end of an era. A beautiful albeit difficult era. 'Can we hug you, doc?' I entreated. He leaned down to my wheelchair to fit comfortably in my left-handed hug.

I often wonder how it must have felt for my family. I had a lot to keep me busy. My server was going haywire, but their time was dotted with so much uncertain waiting, and this for a long stretch of time. It must have felt like a marathon. As I said my thanks to Dr Lui the night before my discharge, he said he was not even the first person on the list to thank. I was honestly befuddled. 'Your family,' he prompted. They were with me every gloomy, boring day at the hospital, trailing after me for every therapy session. Such was their love. It was enveloping.

I honestly don't know how I could have endured my experience. I didn't consciously fight for my life like I needed it. It honestly didn't feel like my battle. I felt like the battleground. Someone else was palpably fighting for me. As a lawyer, I distinctly felt that someone appealed for me up there. Someone was unequivocally on my side. When I was powerless to make my case, someone so obviously intervened for me when I didn't ask Him to.

Someone I deeply admire and respect once posited to me that while Jesus was undoubtedly a kind and amazing human being, he wasn't a marvel in that several yogis who lived before him had escaped death. Deathlessness was a known thing in the world outside mine; I was just an ignorant babe. I kept shut whenever he brought this up, having no worthy refuting argument. I didn't want to be this legalistic, fixed, unreasonable conversationalist about faith. And then it hit me like lightning one day. It wasn't about deathlessness. It was precisely about His death. He was endowed with the capacity to live above death, yet He chose to die as humanly as possible. He was my intervenor, my holy sacrifice that gave me access to the Father. It was the only way I could have survived.

Justice is quite plainly me dying at thirty-five, at the supposed height of my life. Mercy is allowing me to live through my stroke. Grace is giving me a chance to get my life back. My family wheeled me outside the elevator doors of the hospital. It was bright outside. I had not seen the outside for so long; it was almost glistening. It was old yet it was new, as if we were both reluctant to meet each other. We crossed the street to our new apartment across the hospital. There were huge ceiling-to-floor windows overlooking a residential street beside which my wheelchair was parked. Welcome back, I said to myself. *Welcome back.*

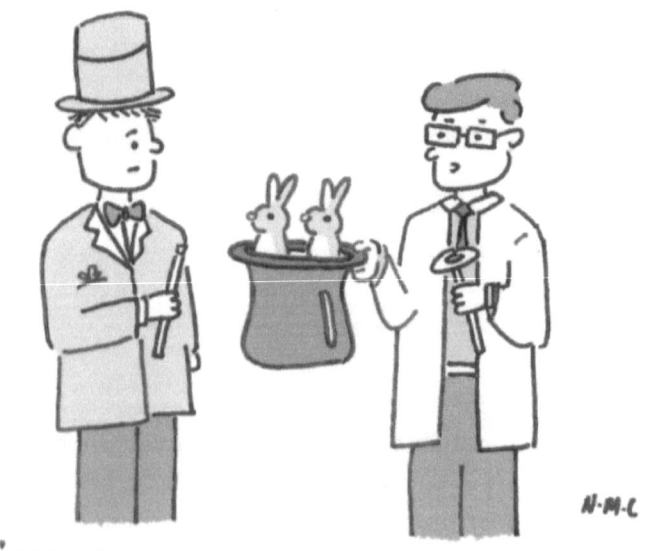

" *MY PATIENTS EXPECT ME TO PERFORM MAGIC TOO* "

A cartoon by Dr Nicolle Marie Chew, used with permission

Part 3

36

I wish I could tell you that things got better from here, but they didn't. I was no longer in the hospital, but I was in a smaller prison. When everything was free and open, I found how trapped I was in my own body.

People were jittery around me, bearers of their own trauma from my experience. They were coping at their own pace, and I had to deal with how fast or slow they healed. It wasn't just my discharge I was dealing with. They were being discharged too, from the nine weeks in the Philippine and Singapore hospitals.

It was a period of a myriad of adjustments. I was awake well before anyone else, well before the sun was up. I looked at Kim at my side. How could I wake her? She was exhausted beyond measure. When I slept, she took the chance to catch up on her work. It was a gruelling schedule—these past months. She was my primary caregiver and now with me sick, primarily handled our business. I lay beside her awake, leaving myself to my thoughts. Once morning broke and my eyes opened, I didn't want to close them again, afraid that the day would pass me by.

I felt helpless and dependent for everything. I felt like a log you could roll over in bed. The extensor tone in my leg had increased then. My right leg shot out straight even when someone tried to bend it. Bending it was like bending an aluminium pipe. I felt like there was an iron rod that was planted in my back connecting everything that my body moved only as one heavy lump. In the beginning of the night, I was gingerly placed on the bed, as if asking my body parts to dutifully take their place. I would be in that position until morning.

I still couldn't control my bladder well, so I always wanted to go potty in the middle of the night. I had to wake my mom and sister who would switch on the light so I could get feedback from my eyes. I would then put on my splint, my shoes, sit on the commode, and press my bladder to stimulate it to go. The whole process was laborious. I silently moaned thinking of the steps to get one thing done. But I had to account for everything. I couldn't count on others to remember everything for me. I had to be three steps forward in mind. I then realized, to be absent-minded is the privilege of the normal.

I had to let go of a lot of things. If my caregiver was not as neat as I wanted her to be, if my dad collected the smallest articles to repurpose at home, I had to learn to turn my back and refuse to see the clutter. I literally willed myself to look at one side of the wall only so all the clutter wouldn't bog my broken brain. I understood clearly my new diminished level of agency. Being dependent on everything, I tried to be as uncomplicated as possible. It was not difficult. You would find that things you would have found important to lug around in daily life were not important enough to bring to the hospital. My pared-down life could fit in my backpack. As I listened in on my surroundings while seated immobile on my wheelchair, I found that I was the least complicated person in the room. Because everything came easy, normal people liked to complicate everything. There was a negotiation for every course of action. I trained myself to hear past their words. I needed to declutter my life.

It was a new phase of my life. The world was the same, but I was different. I got to live it in another dimension. I had to traverse the short distance between our apartment and the out-patient Rehabilitation Centre or *rehab* as we fondly called it. On the way, I had to cross a link bridge, a mall, and ride through several elevators. It was a different worldview. I was brought literally down to the level of babies in carriages and toddlers who could hardly keep their inquiring expressions from their faces as they clutched their mothers' hand. Some retreated to the back of the elevator, unsure of what exactly I was. I was neither an adult nor a child.

Adults gave way to me, opening doors for me, letting me in through elevator doors first. Strangers from the apartment started giving me things like sticky rice from Indonesia. I couldn't have thought to give a random person a gift, but I guess those barriers are removed by virtue of your handicap. By their pity, it was acceptable to be kind.

Because I was so young and in a wheelchair, even adults couldn't keep their gazes away from me. *She's got her whole life ahead of her*, I could almost hear their sympathetic thoughts. I bought a baseball cap to avoid their penetrating stares and feel a tad more invisible.

I finally made my way for the first time to out-patient rehab. I was nervous like a girl in a new class would be, getting familiar with something completely new. Looking back, I realize now how pivotal that moment was. I was meeting my long-term therapists for the first time. On them depended how well I would learn to move in the future. I was now on my third month from the stroke. The golden period, as they say, is just six months from the stroke. It is the critical period when they say one has to recover the movements before they are lost forever.

My physiotherapist, Siva, a serious, kind man rightfully exuded the aura of the chief by his posture. He was learned, calm, and professional. My parents were adamant that I have physiotherapy and occupational therapy sessions twice a day. He insisted that one session each for physiotherapy and occupational therapy were enough, but my parents wanted to desperately squeeze from me what my body allowed.

I could sense his frustration. Everything was measured through time then. *How many months will rehabilitation take from my life?* One month was fine. Three months was acceptable. Six months seemed too long. He was wary to say how long before I could recover. How did 'recovered' look anyway? To walk with a limp and a walking cane like an elderly person? To get movement on the shoulder and wrist and hopefully my fingers? Was recovery towards a fully functioning human being too much to ask? 'What will happen will happen,' he deftly said.

37

My dad took longest to heal. He would take me to the garden to steal time away with me. While I would be munching on my Cheetos, he would just stare at me, a sort of sticky gaze that I could not peel myself away from. I now understand what my grandmother felt when she was on her deathbed. She said she felt like a goldfish in a fish tank. She would wake up in the middle of the night and incredulously exclaim, 'Oh, you're still there.' I know I was their greatest concern, but I did not expand in love by the beholding. I shrunk like a peanut. Are we not taught not to stare from the youngest age? Yet here I was for the whole world to stare at. I couldn't take saccharinity. I was fighting my toughest battle.

I would have crying bouts once every month near my period. My patience would wane, fatigue would set in, and in a matter of seconds, I would lose it. My cry was like a raging river that breaks through a dam unexpectedly. I had no filter. The floodgates to my emotions would open, whether I liked it or not. There was no hiding what I felt. It lay transparently on my shoulder.

It was more like a wail. It ran so deep. I didn't know where it came from. I wasn't particularly sad. The Prozac well-masked my pain that I didn't quite know it, but I couldn't avoid it once a month. It rang clear and spoke only truthfully. By the depths of its pain, I knew my unconscious could only be telling the truth. It was my pain, naked and unadorned and demanding to be acknowledged. It was like a high-pitched hiss that broke out until the wells of my being were satisfied. It was embarrassing to have it the night before and go to rehab the next morning with puffed eyes as if nothing had happened. People expected me to go on living the same way, but a bridge had been burnt, and I had to grieve it.

People also felt the liberty to touch me. If they touched me while walking, I could feel where their hands had been as a constant input on my walking. I couldn't shake off the sensation of their touch until much later. I didn't like to be touched. I felt trapped enough in my own body which didn't feel like my own. I didn't want to be touched before the stroke. Neither did I want to be touched after. My sickness didn't erase all hurts and resentment before the stroke that gave one license to touch me, as if a giant eraser starting everything again from the beginning. I was the same person trapped in an utterly debilitating body, continuing my life, albeit in a disfigured form. I may have had the same needs as a child from the outside, but I was a grown woman inside.

I understand there were things my family had to go through in order to survive the ordeal. My mom would create fireworks with her hands hoping to make me smile, as one would do with a newborn. I was treated like a child, but that was all she could muster at the time. I once told my dad to do things aware that he was doing it for others and not for himself. I didn't like his caressing me at every turn, but he needed to do that for himself, unbeknownst to him. Kim so desperately wanted me to get better that she devoted my practically every waking moment to exercise. My legs were like tight rubber, but she bore them as if they were marshmallows. She would stretch my limbs during morning meditation and sleep over my wrinkled hand at night to keep it straight.

I wished people could pick up my pace, but the truth was they could only march to their own. I wanted so much for people around me to resume their own lives, to carry their own weight, but I had to give them room to grieve. They saw that I lost much, and until they could come to terms with the new me, with a lot of human deficits, they were broken. I had caused them to be broken vessels, and they had to find a way to rebuild themselves. As for me, it was easy to come to terms with the crippled me. I had no choice but to wake up to my new reality. I did not have time to wallow in my own demise. I was busy swimming myself ashore. Everyone was grappling with my sickness in their own way. I was just in the middle of it.

38

There is something to be said about independence: how it makes you. All my life, I've made choices that define who I am, but when I had the stroke, I lost all that. When I first had weakness on my left, I couldn't walk to the toilet, so I had to use a bedpan then a diaper pad. I had to shed my embarrassment very quickly because I had no choice. I couldn't function basically if I didn't spread my legs, naked to accept help from strangers.

Of course, at first, every encounter felt like being stripped of my clothing at every first meeting. Even with people I was familiar with, I was unprepared to be that dependent, to be that unwrapped and vulnerable. It was like being back as a baby, but with an adult mind, my experience being coloured with adult concerns.

I needed a caregiver after my discharge. I was free of all the nurses, but that only meant someone had to replace their care. I was overwhelmed with all the adjustments I needed to make. I was not used to a personal carer 24/7, but it had to be done. I had to prepare myself for these eventualities because it was the only way forward.

The week after my discharge, I met my caregiver, Mai-Mai. She had flown in from the Philippines. She was stocky and sturdy enough to carry me. She stayed with me all day. If I had any free time to myself, she would tinker with my hands and feet, place a hot pack here and there. We would be in the garden, killing time, enjoying the sunshine, except I wasn't really. I was forever thinking of what she could do while I was doing personal things.

I was uneasy to have another human being watch my every move. I wanted her to be preoccupied with something as I did my own thing.

My own thing. That was something I had to dispel as a notion quickly if I was to keep sane. I was closely watched at the dinner table, four sets of eyes anticipating my every hopefully successful swallow. My sushi and any hope of eating it like a normal person disappeared when it was broken down into pieces, looking more like leftover disparate pieces of vegetable and fish than the gastronomic delight it was. I felt unable to enjoy a simple meal with everyone hanging in suspense at my every swallow.

Despite the agonizing discomfort, I, of course, understood. It was too early to demand to be like a normal human being. I remember the feeling that one can go any time simply by a choke. It was an extremely sobering and surprisingly light moment. It made me see the present easily. My vulnerability was exposed. I lived step by step.

I remember the happy reunion I had with my cousins, Louie and Monica, when they visited me in Singapore a week after my discharge. We decided to get all our favourites in the food court and have a feast at home. We went crazy at the food court. We got sushi, lasagne, and tiramisu and set them in a spread before us. In the midst of sharing huge laughs and chewing my spinach lasagne, a leaf caught in my throat. I could not breathe. My panic registered in my eyes. Kim read my expression and shrieked. My mom, sister, and caregiver lunged at me, pressing my chest with their arms, attempting a Heimlich manoeuvre. I coughed up the spinach that blocked my throat. In silence, we all solemnly breathed a sigh of relief. We had survived more than just a meal. With my wobbly left hand, I raised a glass to my lips, sipping water to calm myself down. Even taking something to calm myself down was a gamble. Drinking water was the hardest thing to do.

I found solace in two things. It sprung up inside me like a lightbulb moment. I knew I had to purge myself of my wants in order to create space for myself where others had crowded in. I wanted so badly to just drop everything and watch a show on Netflix, but there was no *just watching* now. There was no solitude as I knew it now. I had to make use of my idle time. Kim would drag my arms open as I watched a film, hoping to insert some passive exercise in my leisure time. Sometimes, if I was running on empty, it would ruin me. I wanted to know rest other than sleeping, but desperation can be pervasive, and you need to work with it. I told my therapist that the eyes never lie. When my soul demanded rest so desperately that I broke down when exercise found its way into my leisure time—no matter how passive—I saw defeat in Kim's eyes. She succumbed to my request but only at the expense of a part of herself. I knew then that my fight and, consequently, my triumph was not mine alone.

I cried freedom, but what I understood as freedom enslaved me. For the first time, I was able to have a bird's eye view of my life. It was like seeing the forest when all I ever had a glimpse of were the trees. How deceptive of a concept freedom was. It felt like a movie, revealing a riveting, unexpected twist only in the end.

I also found that I could only truly be alone when I was being pushed on a wheelchair on the way to rehab. It was ten minutes of unspoken solace. For that period of time, my soul recharged in a way only I knew how.

If there was something I grieved for after the stroke that relentlessly visited and revisited me during my recovery, it was losing my independence. *Where do I place the self when my deficits are clamouring for all of my attention?* I was more than the sum of my parts, but it was hard to make someone see that, not when every medical journal said repetition was the key to getting better. I was not made for all movement. I was not mechanical. It was not just the deficient me that survived. Something whole in me survived too.

I understood my predicament. I knew I only had to be tough for a little while. I knew my hard work was only for my own good in the future, that this was only for the meantime. But the meantime was all I was sure I had.

39

I was unsparing after the stroke. I didn't hold back on what I wanted to say. I felt I earned a certain credibility after going through my ordeal. I wanted to strike while the iron was hot. I suddenly could say things I could not have dared to say before the stroke. I felt like I had no time to waste to swim in the same pond I had swum in before the stroke. *Iron sharpens iron*, the Bible read. I was like a cutting blade with all good intentions. My mouth spewed aphorisms like I could not contain it. Mimi joked that I liked to give my 'lectures' at the breakfast table. I knew those lectures were one-sided. Nobody dared then to expose my own faults; no one dared to make me cry.

I fasted a lot after the stroke, and I was filled with a discipline I did not know before I had the stroke. I would choose something to fast for every week. Whenever I would be tempted, I would, like a good soldier, dismiss the temptation. I had a strong inclination not to shortchange God. *Do not cheat God,* I would tell myself. I would not allow myself to break from the path I had promised to take.

I had a strong inclination towards anything original. I was in awe of what my body could do. I figured that if something in our system could go awry, only something in our system could cure it. I viewed original design as superior above all else. I would wheel into a store and get the best type of everything.

It didn't make sense to me to withhold something from myself because there was a better time for it. There was nothing better to invest in but myself. I didn't know about tomorrow. Today was all that mattered to me.

40

Adjusting to riding the wheelchair took some time. It was a complete submission to hands not my own in literally driving my fate. When I got discharged, my family had to get used to pushing my wheelchair. Suddenly, there was the mass of me to consider when turning corners, entering doorways, climbing uphill. They couldn't be as nimble as they used to be. I had to learn to be patient while they learned to navigate their new space wheeling me around. I would fear bumping into or coming too close to an oncoming person. I would feel helpless trying to avert that disaster so I would raise my good hand to show that I wanted to stop but could not. I wasn't exactly one entity any more. My 'I' was divorced into splints that made the whole of me.

We would take walks around the city on my wheelchair. We felt the need to take advantage of Singapore's generous sidewalks that were not available back home. It was only in Singapore that I could 'walk' the streets. There were many handicapped people who lived lives on their own, waiting at traffic stops and roaming through pedestrian sidewalks in their motorized wheelchairs all by themselves. That was how much the city cared for them. Yet despite the evenly paved sidewalks and considerate ramps everywhere, I still felt every bump and crack and stone on the ground. I felt it hurtle my neck and my hip, sometimes with considerable force.

Still, we managed to go a few places, with my family taking turns to push me. Sometimes, they would prepare themselves to sprint if we were going uphill. I thank my family that they never made me feel like excess baggage. There is a selfless devotion required to care for the sick. My sickness demanded so much from the people I love.

41

I never thought I would be one to go through with it. It wasn't even in my reverie. But when you've got limited options, nothing seems too absurd.

His clinic was in a small annex of his house. There were two small beds separated by a curtain, and the air reeked of smoke that permeated every article in the room. I was more curious than frightened when I first stepped into his clinic. I climbed clumsily onto one of the beds. He said his needle was finer than the needle ordinarily used in injections so I should feel no pain. He poked needles on my feet, my hands, my head, and my face. I braced myself for that second when the needle would pierce my skin, but the moment was negligible. It felt like a small ant bite in the great scheme of things. He then put small metal pliers on the head of the needles and ran electricity through them. The ordeal didn't end there. He put what he called *moxi* or *moxa,* rounded ground mugwort leaves, atop the needles. Then to my horror, he took a lighter and burned them as they floated precariously like clouds on top of the needles. I winced as the lighter hovered over the needles on my face. Sometimes, because I had less sensation in my right, the ash from the moxa would burn through my shirt. My sensors were defective, but the minor burns were the least of my troubles. I was trying not to sneeze or laugh when the acupuncturist lighted the moxa over my nose. I was stopping a volcano from erupting all over my face.

I had multiple bouts with that acupuncturist until one day, while practicing walking around my apartment's corridors, a neighbour in crutches chimed jokingly, 'Do you need to borrow my crutches?' He seemed to be genuinely concerned about my case. 'I have a friend who does acupuncture. I have seen miracles happen before my own eyes,' he offered enthusiastically. So the next day, my Pakistani neighbour, Sajeda, and I piled ourselves in a taxi and made our way to a residential area where the new acupuncturist's clinic was located. Henry, the neighbour in the crutches from Hong Kong, came to translate for us. We were like a couple of international kids on a field trip.

He was a bald, elderly man with a long, snowy white beard that ran down until his navel. He looked every bit like a kung fu master. If acupuncturists had a poster boy, it was him. He wore a factory uniform smudged permanently with grease.

There were tables in front of his store where people gathered to get a quick prickly fix to their minor ailments. The atmosphere was neighbourly, as if it was commonplace to get a needle sting in the middle of tea break. He would swiftly strike the people's necks with his short needles as they would chat carelessly over the day's affairs. We would watch stunned as he would pin the needles through clothes and even sneakers. I gulped down nervously as I clambered onto one of the beds at the back of his store. It was my turn.

He took out his needles. They were of varying widths and lengths. Some looked as long as the diameter of my thigh. 'Bigger needles for the tougher muscles,' Henry explained. The new guy spoke no English and may have doubtfully heard of sanitation (in the Western sense). He poked, rather shoved, needles in my arms, legs, feet, toes, head, forehead, at the corner of my eyes, on the side of my lips, and near my navel, supposedly to give me warmth. He was as fast as lightning that I had neither the time to brace myself nor to react. He dished out needles like they were soiled plates to be washed. He poked a needle diagonally right between my eyes, which left me wondering where the body conjured space inside me for the length of his needle. His acupuncture hurt like hell, by far the most painful procedure in my journey. I would shriek, twist, and writhe in pain, as current ran through my leg. He was precise that way. His needle seemed to connect to an invisible nerve in my body. I thought I felt current with the first guy, but I undoubtedly felt a tidal wave of a current with this one. I always prided myself at having a very high pain tolerance, but having needles twisted in place while being poked inside my body without an ounce of pain-killing medication was just too much to take. He then ran a giant roll of moxa all over my body before putting me under very hot infrared lights. I was like a pig roasting in an oven.

My mother couldn't help making pained sounds at every poke that I couldn't help but laugh. The laugh reverberated all over my body. It was a dose of inconvenient laughter. My Western doctor of a sister struggled to watch the procedure, lamenting that acupuncture was too much of a stretch for her and that I should just trust my Western-prescribed physiotherapy.

The new guy would let me turn on the bed and poke more needles with me lying face down. We wanted him not to touch the neck, but good luck on getting a word through him. He distrusted Western doctors. So, despite our protests, he shoved two needles deftly at the side of my neck. It was so fast. It was like a sleight of hand. I once asked him how he could remember all the meridian points in the body. He said he didn't; I wouldn't know if he was poking in the right place anyway. Har-dee-har-har.

Through all these torments, the acupuncturist was a very amiable, funny guy who may have been a kung fu master in his past life. He gave out pears when I was done with his torture. He always gave me a coin to hold as I seemed to be always clutching something. My fingers were always curling. He was like an amused grandfather who genuinely wanted me to get well. He had already stopped acupuncture, had acupuncturists working for him, and was perfectly content working at the factory he owned, but he resurfaced for me to do some charity. The people in his store remarked and even cried at how lucky I was that he was treating me.

The acupuncturist prescribed foods to take. *Don't take these, they're cold. These are hot; they're fine.* I once asked Yi Yang, my friend in Singapore who grew up in China, how in the world I was to determine if a food was hot or cold. She said that she grew up knowing these things. To make discussions quicker, she handed me a bag of fruits permissible for me to eat at the next session. The acupuncturist also prescribed bags of herbs for me to soak in three times a day and powdered medicine contained in generic white bottles with no labels. We wanted to check if the powder he prescribed would not interfere with the drugs my Western doctors gave me, so we asked him for its mysterious contents. Well, they remained mysterious. Traditional Chinese medicine allegedly existed since ancient times while Western medicine allegedly was borne in the civilized world. There was no point of comparison. It's either you believed it or didn't.

Well, truly with no pain, there was no gain. I gathered bruises at the side of my lips, in my eyebrow and arms, looking like someone who got a beating in all the unusual places. But the night I had my first session, I felt my right foot flatten on the ground. By the third session, I felt my face start to ease up, my lips straighten. In the following days, my hands always wound in a tight fist significantly opened, revealing my palm. My appetite increased. I ate greedily after his session, as if rewarding myself for the mental toughness I had to have before seeing him each time. I began to sleep as deeply as I had right after the stroke. I took two-hour naps in the middle of the afternoon. The kung fu master turned out to be a jolly gift beneath a porcupine of a disguise.

42

I first met Siva the weekend after my discharge. I had then thought that I needed to make another adjustment, just when things were getting stable. I had loved my therapist in the hospital. He was my road map to how to live this new life. To say the least, I was reluctant to meet my new outpatient therapist.

The first time I met him, he said there was nothing that fascinated him any more. After twenty-seven years of service, he had seen everything. That night I lay around in my bed, thinking of fascinating trivia to throw at him. *What would throw him off his feet?* Well, it turned out that he was unfamiliar with the word, 'trivia'. He thought it was some restaurant, and my first attempt at establishing rapport failed, but we found common ground soon enough, and rehab soon came not to be a place to pass routine, but a place to look forward to.

Rehab was a mix of mental, physical, psychological, and spiritual therapy. One time, Kim told me that she noticed he used a certain approach when dealing with me. He would put a chair in front of me and ask me to bend forward to stand. The chair was supposed to give me some mental comfort that something would catch me if I were to fall. It spoke volumes about my confidence in the early days, but more than that, he was earning my trust.

Siva never treated me like a child, which seemed to be the instinctual reaction of others when dealing with a stroke patient, nor did he simply let me do the motions. He let me get my bearings, allowed me time to gather my inner self before

I executed his action. He gave me what I needed, at a time when I badly needed it. He made time wait for me, impossible then as it may have seemed.

* * *

Siva never failed to throw witticisms when he had the opportunity in between sessions. One day, Siva bandaged my right leg and taught me my first steps. He looked into my eyes and said, 'I want you to walk, but I don't see the desire to walk within you yet.' Another time, he opened *The Body Keeps the Score*, a book that I had given him, and pointed to a part he had underlined. 'I don't know how many times I have to drill this in your head. The brain has to rewire in order to fire.' It made me pause to consider my motivation. *Did I to want to walk enough when this world I knew now offered me so much more?* Everyone wanted and rooted for me to be normal, but I was not convinced I wanted to be. Sitting on a wheelchair meant I got to drop my self-consciousness. Heck, I donned a neon orange luggage strap for a belt. I wore a disposable plastic apron even when eating in public. After that, I couldn't have cared how I looked. Still, everyone wanted me to walk, so four times a day I braced myself for physical and occupational therapy every time the elevator doors to rehab opened. I practically spent my whole day there.

Siva appeared to be a very wise, evolved person, and I often wondered how one could be evolved that way. He had a peace and giddiness about everyday life that I never saw before. One day, he told me that he was going on a cruise. I asked him, 'To where?' He stopped and thought to himself for a moment before going completely agog. 'I think the cruises here don't go anywhere. They just sail around.' That took me aback. I thought that he probably didn't want to tell me where he was going. Months later, as I knew him better, it became clear that he really didn't seem to know or care where he was going. He came back showing us photos of how he surfed fake waves and slid down giant slides on board the ship. In one of our sessions, he mused that it boggled him why people didn't seem as enthusiastic as him about his experience. I gave it a thought. Perhaps people were always impatiently more concerned about the destination, and he was just all about the ride. I could never have in a million years put my stroke in my calendar. I had to learn to be along only for the ride.

* * *

Siva's sessions were extremely cerebral. He demanded every ounce of me when we were on. If I moved my foot an inch more than how much he said, he would ask me why I did the same. 'Never assume,' he would admonish. He ran a tight ship.

Every day, he gave me a mountain to scale. It was normal for everyday people, but it was a mountain to me. 'Think before you execute an act,' he would advise. Sometimes, he would see me doing a motion but never really understanding what we were doing the motion for. 'No recognition, no awareness,' he would mutter, prompting me to do an action again. I wondered how he must have known that my understanding was incomplete. With an incomplete brain, I was at the boundaries of what my brain could do. I knew I had reached my edge when my conscious brain would just let go. I would lose any control over it and release uninhibited laughter. Nothing was funny. I was just exhausted beyond my limits.

Every step was a test of my balance. 'Walking is just keeping your balance at every step,' Siva would say. I couldn't afford to fall. My arm raised at my elbow stiffly while walking, as if perpetually raised for the teacher to call me. I walked like a zombie, my mind so busy at how to execute every step that I gave blank stares. *Soft knees. Mount your hip on your bad knee. Trust your bad knee and swing your good leg.* I ran a mantra in my head. Since everybody was acquainted with me in rehab, the therapists around would kindly give me their input on my walking, as if I were on perpetual evaluation.

Siva would simulate a sandy surface, an uphill climb, and wobbly ground made from cushioned balance pads in the gym. He would push me hard unknowingly at my back and sides to perturb me. He would deliberately try to outbalance me to bring out a reflex. I would fall behind and calmly let my body to a free fall, like a buoy hanging from a crane. My fear sensors were deactivated. I did not know that I should save myself. When I did eventually learn the need to save myself, the reaction I needed from my body took long to conjure. I knew that bringing my hips to the centre and bending my knees would save myself, but there was a delay in my brain commanding my body to do just that. It was like having a smart enough controller but a poor executor. Still, Siva would challenge me to take the train, stand while it braked and moved, while it was still a challenge for me to remain standing. (Good luck trying that exercise in my own country.) Siva tested what I could do. He taught me early on that I was only as vast as my brain would recognize.

I bombarded Siva with tons of questions. He was always indulgent with me and generous with his time, as long as it helped me. More often, our conversations swerved to the existential. He never dismissed my random, out-of-the-blue, funny but honestly curious questions. I wanted to learn as much as I could from the man.

He never wanted to call me by my nickname. He wanted the power of my full name to dress me. *Warlike. Fighter. Warrior.* That's what my name meant. I never expected something so delicate and urban carried with it such a sturdy, almost military meaning. I wondered whether the moment I was named, I was being prepared by the universe for this moment that was to come. My whole life seemed to boil down to this one, defining moment. I needed the force of my name to arm me with what I had to find yet within myself.

I count myself lucky to have found rehab such a rehabilitating space both for my body and soul. Siva and my stroke gave me what I thought was beyond me. He taught me more than walking.

43

My philosophy teacher once said we are good at passing by people. We pass them on the trains, on the way to work, while getting a coffee. But you can't do that in rehab. You look at a guy strapped to his chair, who can barely shut his one eye and get his neck to carry his head, and you know a part of his story. It is a story that stares you in the face and lingers at the back of your mind before you can pass it by.

There was a guy in such a bad state in rehab. He always kept his head down low. He had one eye bigger than the other so he always looked surprised. He always wore a black cap and a sporty black shirt, as if that would fade him from view. His glasses had tape across them, demarcating what was reality and what was mere duplication. He was in such bad shape that I couldn't look at him. He suffered from a bad brainstem stroke. If it could have gone any worse, he would have been bedridden. I was staring at what I could have become had my arteries broken further.

Because the brainstem deals with the primitive brain and his was debilitatingly incapacitated, he could not talk. Meanwhile, the rest of us 'classmates' in the gym chattered in our own slurred way. We chatted over and above him. I tried not to look at him so that it didn't appear as if I was purposely excluding him. I assumed he could hear and follow our conversations as he did his therapy. His broken brain was capable of higher cognitive functions; he just could not use it for the most basic of functions. He stunned me. I was frozen by his deficit.

I recalled my first day with Siva when my mouth could hardly move to mouth what I wanted to say. He asked me what I ate for breakfast. I immediately looked at Kim to respond. I was used to people not understanding me clearly, so I looked at her to answer for me. 'No, what did YOU have for breakfast?' he insisted. In an instant, he gave me back to myself. I had almost forgotten I existed separately and distinctly from others. He was just like Mr Lim, the special needs driver, who always made it a point to look me in the eyes at the back mirror to ask me how the air conditioning was at the back. Or Mr Ong, the other special needs driver, who liked to take the longer route to our apartment so I could catch a glimpse of the touristy places, making me feel like I was more than my sickness. Or Dr Lee who talked about his favourite food court finds at the mall across my dreary room in the hospital, as if everything was just as it should be. They all gave me back to myself piece by piece. I hoped to let him in on the conversation even if just to include him silently.

We were a cast of characters in rehab. There was Simon. He spelled independence in a way I didn't know how. He would wheel himself into rehab by puttering his feet on the ground, reminding me of Fred Flintstone driving his stone car by his feet. He would have his head down low and his brows furrowed. He had a severe vestibular problem that in the early days would make him puke as he would turn to his sides doing therapy. He came so close to dying that he was comatose for two months. No one thought he would come out of his experience alive and walking, yet here he was in rehab tying his own shoestring, cycling, and beating his own record in the gym. I am glad I met him early in my recovery. He showed me that you can be happy with the crumbs you're given. You can be joyful in the in-between, in the increments.

Then there was this quiet figure of a mother steadfastly accompanied by her teenage son. She came from another rehabilitation centre that saw a dead-end in her. She would position herself on the bar in front of the mirror and look at her leg and foot. It was the only way she could command them to move. She could not feel them. With an incapacitated brain, she had to teach herself where her foot was and command it to take a step. I dared not look at the mountain she had to climb.

There was Ananda with a right-sided stroke much like mine who could not talk. He was sullen, as I imagine I would be, if I went through what I was going through and yet not be able to talk to anyone about it. He learned his alphabet—a grown man, probably head of his business empire and relegated back to kindergarten. Every time he'd learn a new word, he'd practise it on us. 'Bye' or 'Hi', he'd bellow in the gym. We were like proud parents hearing the first words come out the mouth of a child. Our colleague, previously mute, could now talk! Our milestones were now measured vastly differently.

There was Madame Kho who looked A-okay on all her scans, but, obviously, there was something awry inside her brain as she could not walk straight. For the life of her, she could not treat what she had because she didn't know what was wrong with her. What a sprightly character, she was. She still went to Finland and Vietnam despite her condition. Any normal person would have thought it acceptable to cancel a leisure trip because of a serious condition, but thank God, the thought did not occur to her.

Then there was this grandfather whose left side of the head seemed bludgeoned by an axe. The left side of his head seemed lopped off, such that his head looked like a misshapen egg or slime that hadn't fully settled to its final shape. He was always in high spirits, chatting up therapy assistants like nothing shocking had happened to him. *Perhaps they got a part of his skull and left only his brain?* We didn't dare ask what happened to him. He didn't seem to care. He just cycled his way through gaping stares of people who had to learn to straighten them out after a while. They got old.

There was this teenager who had just come out from a debilitating yet successful surgery. She was air-lifted from

Myanmar. News was that she could walk and she could talk. She was as good as new, except she wanted to give up on her new state of life. She didn't eat. She was uncooperative and even hostile with the doctors and nurses. One day, I saw a pretty young lady hunched, walking slowly but steadily with her mom in the hallway. She was clutching the handlebars at the side to help her walk safely. She was walking, not even hobbling. It was her! She had come out of her pit. What a joy! I felt like cheering her on, except she didn't know me. She was preceded by her surgery and reputation.

There was Madame Lim, who had brought herself to the hospital when she felt a sudden weakness in her limbs. When she got to the hospital, all of her body from neck down was paralysed. She was all business when she came to rehab. Siva would point to her, saying what having done one's homework looked like (obviously pointing out that I had not done my own). She was a picture of a malleable brain. At her age, everyone did not expect much from her, but she defied all odds and surprised us with her walking between the handlebars.

Finally, there was this neurologist who sauntered into rehab. He looked positively stern as he crossed the room to occupy the bed opposite mine. There was a quiet in the room as the 'populace' felt the gravity of his presence. Everyone felt the irony of the situation. The doctor just got discharged from the hospital after a stroke. I could not look straight doing my exercises from my bed, or I would be staring right at him. I felt his steady gaze follow my passive movements. His wife couldn't keep the inquiring expression off her face, as if entering a playground previously hidden from her. A few sessions more and the good doctor became enveloped in our fold. He would watch me doing my exercises and marvel at Siva's latest creative neurological challenge for me. I would share with him socks that spoke silly witticisms, never imagining a moment in my normal life that I could give a neurologist one.

We were like a class no one wanted to be part of. We were like the cast of *One Flew Over the Cuckoo's Nest*, Asian version. I don't remember having such genuine encounters as in my stint in rehab. I saw the characters in that tiny gym more closely. We didn't have the normal concerns. We had been bludgeoned by life, paid a closer visit by death, and everyone knew that there was simply no use acting all fine and perfect. No one could help leaving rehab changed.

* * *

There was a young woman with her husband who always occupied the bed next to mine in rehab. It was inevitable that we would become friends.

One day, I went to the basement floor of our building to get some food, and there she was being wheeled by her husband. Being my normal busybody self, I waved a friendly hello while she looked confused as a squirrel, obviously not recognizing me.

When we found ourselves back in rehab, waiting for our appointments, she finally figured out who I was and wheeled herself forward. She then went through a detailed and impassioned account of what happened to her. There was only one problem. I could barely get a word of what she was saying. She had such a small voice, and her speech was so slurred that she was barely understandable. She was inaudible and incomprehensible.

To act like a decent human being, I politely asked for her name. And the cat was finally out of the bag. We could not understand each other. Only blank stares registered on our faces. We could not form one decent conversation because we would trail off after, 'What is your name?'

We tried to make polite conversation whenever we bumped into each other in rehab, getting only 10 per cent of what the other says, but all is well. We were as close as any slurred friends could come by.

* * *

I wrote feverishly after the stroke. I wrote about all my qualms until I ran dry. It was a way to relieve my brain of chatter. In a way, I needed that empty brain for my recovery. I never successfully attempted to chronicle my affairs before the stroke. I just knew I had to write to relieve my brain of the noise that constantly plagued it. I began to address my letters to a familiar face in rehab. We were in the hospital together and shared the same doctor. He was a dad led to rehab by his downtrodden yet hopeful family. He stood out to me because his family stayed by his side. There were many led every day by their caregivers. After the initial shock wears off, the family usually wears off too, but his family stayed. This made him easily distinguishable. I wrote to him shortly after discharge, pouring into my letter what I could only tell him.

June 8

Dear Santos,

I would be remiss to state that it is all happiness after the stroke and that the adjustment ends after the first hospital visit, but it seems that it is a life-long job—the first fever, the first cold, the first stress. Everything is an adjustment. Perhaps Edward says it best. You can control your mind despite the circumstances. And as my friend lovingly puts it, you only have to be tough for a little while, not all the time. At this time, all my brain seems to consciously grasp is that there is no time to waste.

June 9

Dear Santos,

How wonderful to take a breath. Perhaps normal people don't get it. We need to take a breath. Does it seem to you that the brain was focused on physical healing the first three months then on the fourth month, emotions started coming in? I wish I could be free from all emotions. It is much easier not to think. To tell you the truth, having a routine saved my life. It made me not think about what to do the next day. This life is artificial, of course. No one goes through life without a million things in mind.

I felt my experience was so singular that though many flanked at my side, I felt alone. I didn't know who else understood me or who could possibly understand me, that I addressed my letters to him—who probably had no clue who I was. I couldn't fill my journal without writing to him. I couldn't tell my family that I needed a waking minute just for myself when they were desperate for me to get well. I wrote in my journal, *what was I doing getting back to what I was, when I didn't want to get back to it?* The stroke offered me many things I didn't see. It was like my ears slowly popping from a long flight. The world was being revealed to me as a cripple. Suddenly, there was more to the world than walking. I was content to be immobile in my chair.

* * *

I often stopped to think about the other people doing worse than me in rehab. How must it feel to know that you're not getting better? In that situation, where does hope reside? Can hope blossom at all? What if a perpetually ill person were to see me getting better every day in rehab, and those prospects are not available to him or her? Hope grows on you, but can it grow at all in someone suffering a decline? Their hope must be other-worldly. I decided to ask the hard questions to a young therapist covering for Siva one day. He said that for those going downhill, physical therapy is for maintenance. At the point in time that they are in rehab, they are at their physical best. Therapy aims to maintain that state.

I wondered about the people who disappear in rehab. The brainstem stroke guy still appeared for his morning speech therapy when we learned he was set to be admitted in the hospital that afternoon. He was already in a precarious situation out-patient, but the therapists assured us that his admission was not due to a complication but just his over-anxious imagination. When we didn't see him after a couple of weeks, we learned that he was in a bad way in the hospital. His condition had sorely deteriorated. So had his disposition. When I first saw him, he wasn't as bad. He was still cycling at the stationary bike in rehab. But he got hit by a stroke in the same part of the brain two more times. A therapist said that when a part of the brain gets hit time and again, it couldn't heal itself even if it wanted to. She said that it was just a matter of time. It wasn't sayable, but it was understood. Death was lurking nearby. I hoped hard that hope sprung even from a place so desolate. Fall down seven times, get up eight. Isn't that what they say? Maybe that is the province of faith. You don't know what's at the end, but you do it anyway.

44

Though always kind and amiable, my occupational therapist had an air of professionalism about her. If I were friendlier, I was afraid to appear as a busybody. At first, I didn't know what to do with my time with her. The passive range of exercises she performed created a pregnant silence that begged my Filipino self to be filled. It seemed easier to break the ice with my other therapists. I was throwing silly, friendly trivia to them, but not directly at her. Her name was Belle.

Belle worked tirelessly with me, arranging and rearranging her schedule to accommodate me, until I was out of the 'danger zone'. I didn't know what that meant. *To what degree could my fatalistic situation become even more dangerous?*

I stared at my hands. I could not see my palms because my fingers would stiffly curl to cover them. They would sweat incessantly. I never had sweaty hands before the stroke. One month in. Two months in. Three months in. No movement in my arm. My arm was attached to my trunk like a block of ice that had melted and attached to the one beside it. It had to be pulled off my trunk, like a pull rope that one violently tugs at to start a rickety, old engine. Belle bore the weight of my arm every day as she swung it in all directions. She was quiet, maybe silently solemn for the things she could not tell me, trying to be hopefully expectant yet reasonably practical. She was perhaps inwardly gathering the strength to tell me my verdict in the end. Too much time my limbs would spend lifeless would make my brain forget that it had an arm to use in the first place. Learned helplessness would kick in, and my arm would be dead for all intents and purposes.

We persevered in the danger zone, with me never understanding where the zone ended. Ever so slowly, I felt that my brain finally understood the action we were doing. It was just not Belle tugging at my arm. There was me. It was the faintest feeling, but it was undeniably there. *A brain connection. Maybe that's how it felt.* There were movements, nothing but a flicker, all over my body. There was the slightest movement in my pinkie, and I knew it moved. It was good progress from me looking at my arm move and wondering if I had anything to do with it.

I looked at the young man on the bed across me. He was independent and able. He walked to rehab alone, even though he had to pass through a bustling mall to get to the place. I couldn't have imagined myself crossing a place successfully alone with so much distraction. On a tragic vacation and amidst a major holiday, he got his stroke. Resources were scant during the holiday and he did not get the immediate treatment he needed. When he finally did, he was already half-paralysed. His therapist tried to recover function in his limbs, moving them constantly to get a flicker of movement from his muscles. Movement finally came to his shoulder and his elbow, but not his fingers. He looked just like any teenager, except he lost use of his fingers. I asked Belle how his therapist knew that there was nothing to be done to retrieve function in his fingers. How could his therapist know that it was the end of the line for him, that it was time to drop arms and surrender to fate? What if one more passive stroke could bring back function? I did not want to give up for his sake.

One day, Siva was out, and Belle was sitting by the window, perhaps waiting for her next patient. She threw me a piece of trivia and a smile. I heaved a sigh of relief for her and for me. I felt her a comrade in my cause. Mercifully, I guess I was out of the danger zone.

45

We liked to stay in the garden of our apartment sometimes to get some sun, Singapore's heavy rains and interconnected walkways not affording us much. So, when the situation allowed, we just liked to plant ourselves in one of the outdoor chairs of the apartment's garden and enjoy the prickly pinch of the sun on our skin.

Sometimes, we would unpack a breakfast picnic of some toast, cinnamon rolls, avocado, mushrooms, eggs, blueberries, and some cold cuts—a helping from the breakfast buffet they allowed me to take away due to my condition. On Sundays, we would play *Bananagrams* just to pass the time. 'A book, the sun, and time in between—a gift straight to the soul,' I used to say in the bookstore I ran. Now, it had come true. I had all three—a book, the sun, and time in between.

Some days, I would just sit in the garden during my breaks, munching on a little snack before dinner. By the afternoon, the children would come out to swim. I would go there every day and grow familiar with the faces of the children who would come to swim daily. There was that Chinese boy, about nine, who somehow always found himself in the middle of families who were vacationing during the season. He didn't feel himself a tad out of place. There were the two Nordic kid brothers who liked to playfully annoy the Crazy Rich Asian-esque vacationer, sunbathing at the edge of the pool, with the most ludicrous of dance moves.

The kids would swim gracefully underwater. They would never lap. They preferred to be rowdy and exuberant above water, jumping in the pool with their legs under their butts and splashing everyone nearby, running over ledges, and plunging through decorative overflows that were not meant to be swum in.

I, of course, had a front-row seat to all this living as I sat in my wheelchair under the warmth of the afternoon sun. I could see how the children dove and played raucous games underwater, as our apartment pool had this huge transparent section made of glass. I watched as day by day they grew closer to each other. Maybe they started as friendly nameless acquaintances who played water football together until they became the kind of unspoken friends that one meets one magical summer (kids don't exchange e-mails).

I needed to be reminded of that beating, pulsating part of life that made it worth living, that secure feeling that you could do anything because your father was always there watching over you. Where else could the confidence of kids come from? Nurture has not taken root yet. All parts still come from the original maker.

46

Victor Hugo said, 'Be kind for everyone is fighting a different battle.' I understood it when I read it before the stroke. It was a nice quote to put on a tote. I thought inwardly, *we are all fighting a different battle*—but always with four limbs. It was always a presupposition.

One day, I went to the apartment lounge, and there was a family with six-year-old twins being tutored. I couldn't quite make out what was up with them, but something was off. Every day, I saw them as I was having breakfast in the garden. Some days they would swim and make unusually loud squeals and splashes. Then, I finally got it. They were deaf.

There was this other kid in the apartment. He had two caregivers who tutored him every morning. On breaks, a caregiver would blow bubbles for him to chase, probably to throw off his excess energy. He would lackadaisically and unenthusiastically run after them. The exercise seemed more routine to him than fun. Later, I would no longer see him in the garden, although I would still see his caregivers around the apartment. I would later learn from them that the boy was now on nasogastric tube because of too little food intake.

Then there was this old lady who only came out in the afternoons. I don't think I ever heard her talk. She always had her head hung low, and it seemed like she was sleeping even when she wasn't. Her caregivers would chat around her, as she would sit motionless in her wheelchair to get some sun. She and her husband each got a stroke. They've been presumably silent in the apartment for at least three years.

And that was only what was visible. I opened my eyes widely at the mall on the way to rehab. There was a man with a limp. Our concierge in the apartment had a big bulge behind his ears and often disappeared to visit his ailing mother. And how many are behind their doors who could not lift a finger? How many are suffering from peculiar diseases, making them hardly recognizable versions of themselves? How many of us walk with a chip on the shoulder? Be kind indeed for everyone is fighting a different battle.

47

My recovery came in stages. My brain was being returned to me portion by portion. It was amazing to be acutely aware of how my brain restored itself. I had always lived with my head atop my shoulders ever since I was born, but I had been walking with literally half a mind since the stroke.

I had an empty brain. It was solace to swim in such clarity. Every thought seemed to come out of me with a little push of pure air. It was clear as day. There was no second-guessing myself. It was interesting how my thoughts seemed to stop abruptly up until the stroke. Since the stroke, I had no forward thought. It was as if my life as I had known it stopped with it.

I couldn't multi-task. If I wanted to empty my bladder, I had to focus on the task 100 per cent. I couldn't participate in brainstorming and work sessions. It bogged my empty, clear brain. It was a nirvana I knew would not come again. Though in many ways that period was characterized by an unloading of a lot of hurts that enabled me to have a clean slate, that time was precious time when everyone carried the weight of the world for me.

Then the thoughts flooded. I was afraid of them. I was afraid of the seemingly innocuous thoughts that would gnarl their sticky fingers on my brain. I was afraid that when one swam in, the floodgates of my brain would open, and I wouldn't be prepared to meet any of them. But they came, and prepared as I was or not, the period of imagination followed. I couldn't stop daydreaming of the future. It was addictive. I would lie awake with my eyes open as the early morning light streamed in my room and while waiting for everyone to awaken. My brain seemed like it had many rooms to fill, unlike before the stroke when it was cramped.

I was getting reacquainted with my brain. It was like waiting for a long-lost friend to remember who I was. I eagerly awaited a coming back to what I was fully before. My therapist once told me that brain scientists have never found the site of the mind. Truly, I felt like my brain was evolving, but with what did I recognize the evolution? Is it possible that I never lost my mind, but it is somehow retrievable only in full when I recovered my brain? Learning about my brain was a magical thing, and I was right in the thick of it.

48

One Saturday morning, we decided to try, for the first time, swimming or rather wading. We parked my wheelchair at the edge of the kiddie pool and indulged ourselves in two feet of water. No kids could be found at the kiddie pool. They were all gregariously enjoying themselves at the adult pool and jumping off ledges. I looked with amazement at how their tiny legs seemed to effortlessly carry their trunks and how they could saunter off without a care in the world while I had to think about my every step with meticulous care.

There were wide ample steps down the kiddie pool, and I gingerly sat my way down through it. One European girl, about four years old, peeked from the adult pool ledge to watch. My two sisters were in the pool with me, swinging my arms and keeping me afloat. The girl stared at my predicament with captured eyes. I was used to curious staring from children and pitiful glances or deliberate avoidance from adults, so I really didn't mind.

As we went about flailing, I didn't notice that a line of children had formed at the ledge of the adult pool. The little girl may have apparently called her siblings who joined the force. Then they were able to engender a little Chinese girl, decked in all swimming gear, to the staring contest. There was a whole line of them, entranced, as if watching a circus show.

We turned and twisted as my body allowed. Sometimes facing up to the sky and sometimes facing the adult pool while being cradled by one of my sisters, my legs floating loose. It was during one of these instances when I saw the girl's face. It contorted to an unguarded pained look. It was the creeping in of a feeling so alien to herself that she didn't know what to make of it. It took its time as it settled within her. It was coming to understand, for the first time, disability. *How can she run off carelessly and swim through deep waters while I could barely walk?* It was clear-eyed wonder and curiosity mangled with pity. I wished I could etch her face in my memory forever. I could hardly remember the first time I felt things.

It is to be endowed with magical eyes to notice us more than we know. Maybe she'd grow up to be one of those people who know that it is not enough to be occasionally and conveniently kind, who know that their lives exist amidst our suffering, and not apart. Not everybody has that.

49

It is a different feeling of helplessness when you're handicapped. I was in the neurology gym, early for my turn in rehab, when it rang. I stared at my caregiver. She stared at me. The fire alarm rang again. Since we were early, not many were in rehab. I looked around me. No one was panicked, just walking in their normal pace. But this was not the case for me. Becoming handicapped didn't come with a manual. It didn't come with a tutorial, like the way you learned to drive a car for the first time. There was a fire escape, but it consisted of stairs. I could barely move. We were on the eighteenth floor. I presumed that there was a way out that didn't involve the stairs, but it probably involved a rope. I couldn't grip so I was in a pretty dangerous quandary. We asked a therapist if we were to go down. He didn't know what to answer and set about asking about it. It wasn't until we saw Siva that we learned the alarm we heard was part of a fire drill. He said he would be the first to carry me on his back if there was a real fire. If there was a real fire, what was I supposed to do to save myself other than to lie in wait? Being handicapped exposed me to a whole new level of fear.

One day, it was our mother's turn to accompany me to rehab because Kim had contracted COVID-19. I noticed she was coughing occasionally, but I didn't think much of it. I ate lunch with her and even grocery shopped with her. When she kept coughing, we urged her to take a test. She tested positive.

When God teaches you a lesson on dependency, He goes through the whole nine yards. Not long after Kim and my mom contracted COVID-19, my caregiver's mom died. She came to me with red eyes and a glum face after receiving the news. A sullen understanding befell her. She understood she was not going to see her mother. How could she leave me alone when she bathed me, fed me, carried me, watched me at every turn while the others were sick in a foreign country? The whole scenario was complicated by the fact that I couldn't cough. My throat muscles didn't seem to know how to. I didn't know what to expect if ever I did contract COVID-19. *Doesn't it partly manifest in a cough?* I felt my helplessness as a heavy weight.

We eventually came up with a plan that if Kim tested negative the day the virus would have supposedly passed according to health authorities, my caregiver would go home just in time for her mother's burial. We spent the days in suspense, expectant that we would get the virus and yet hoping against hope that we didn't catch it. I did everything with Kim. We slept together. We shared dinners together. She was like my twin in every way. It felt like it was just a matter of time before we got it.

My caregiver and I slept with double masks on. For three days I kept my denture on because I didn't want this stranger (my caregiver whom I had just met) to know that I was missing an incisor. It was intimate information I wanted to keep to myself but was ultimately constrained to reveal. Every day we took a test and held our breaths as a single red line splayed on the results stick. *Negative.* Day after day, with bated breaths, we tested negative— negative until Kim's first day to test negative. We rejoiced. We had made it. She was able to reach home just as her mother's casket was being wheeled out for burial. Just in the nick of time.

I recalled that I had once asked God for patience. *If Solomon had wisdom, let mine be patience.* I didn't know what I was asking for. I had asked pettily. My patience was then being tested, but it was being tried in an ordinary way. It is true, what they say. He doesn't give you patience, only opportunities to be so. Now I know not to take it lightly. *Ask and you shall receive. Seek and you will find.* Am I ready to be asking what I ask for? Now I ask for the courage for Him to use me. I don't know what it will entail but let me fly with wings like an eagle. Let me run and not grow weary.

50

I wouldn't say that I have much of a sweet tooth, but the slew of flavours lining the fridge in the supermarket below rehab was just too much to handle. The ice cream pints were too colourful, and the flavours just begged to be tried.

I worked my butt off on weekdays, lending my arms as if they were not personal property and succumbed to the need to exercise most of the day, but Friday afternoons were sacred to me. I longed to go to the supermarket at the basement to indulge myself. My eyes would scour the aisles greedily. I would spend the time discovering new sauces and mixes and conjuring the menu for the next week. We would take two hours in the supermarket, taking our sweet time amongst familiar aisles. I would try things I would never have the time to try at home. It was a sweet retreat.

The first tub I tried was Dreyer's 'Mint'. It was refreshing and creamy. I would fast the whole week, steering clear of carbs, then reward myself with a bowl on the weekend. There was Häagen-Dazs' 'Green Tea'. It was clean and sophisticated like a grandma wearing pearls. Then there was Ben and Jerry's 'Chewy Gooey Cookie'. It was coconut ice cream specked with brownie and cookie crumble. It was light and decadent with the hint of the East. But the one that took the cake for me was Ben and Jerry's 'Cherry Garcia', recommended by no other than Dr Lee, the unapologetic ice cream connoisseur.[8] It was subtle, smooth, and unexpected. Every flavour (though we hated cherry) fell into place. It was like my sickness, like a chip on the shoulder that fell into place.

* * *

Early into my discharge, my Aunt Mila came to visit me. We decided to do the most touristy thing and go to Gardens by the Bay. It was magnificent. It more than met my expectations. I've been to lauded gardens before, and they always seemed to be on sprawling grounds, cultivating plants that were endemic to the area. But Gardens by the Bay was different. It featured plants from deserts to rainforests, all under one air-conditioned dome. It didn't seem like the plants were floundering either; they were blossoming. The Philippines didn't seem ten times poorer than Singapore. It seemed a hundred times poorer. If Singapore could spend so much money for a lush garden, I guess it had all its more important needs taken care of.

   We decided to have lunch at this traditional Chinese restaurant at the premises. Because it was one of only two accessible restaurants in the area, it was filled with people. The maître d' seemed busy. We asked for two tables. I had just been discharged and couldn't swallow very well. I needed to be seated separately from my cousin who was a master jokester because it was too dangerous for me to laugh while attempting to swallow. My caregiver and I would sit at a table by ourselves and secure an environment conducive for me to eat. The maître d' couldn't get that. People were waiting in line to be able to secure a spot inside. He didn't understand why we needed two tables. He certainly did

---

[8] I gave Dr Lee a sinful traditional chocolate cake to pair with the Cherry Garcia and wholeheartedly apologized for blaming my weight gain on the new brand of laxative.

not need our petty requests at such a busy hour. I was already halfway through the restaurant when the maître d' decided to make the matter more complicated than it seemed. As everybody seemed to argue before me, I decided to just leave the restaurant. End the conversation like that. Spare me a moment as an invalid on my wheelchair in the spotlight and just leave. The maître d' ignored us and chose not to give us two tables. Kim was adamant that we be given our seats and not be treated differently because of the inconveniences of my precarious situation. She said that now she will defend herself every time she was in the right. I would have done the same if I found myself in our situation before the stroke. I would have fought for what's right fervently.

Fr Gregory Boyle said moral outrage is often mistaken for moral righteousness. I was done with the outrage part, but I knew I wasn't letting go of the righteousness. I didn't feel the need to fight, but I didn't feel stripped of my right either. I didn't even feel riled up. I just literally wanted to drop it and go.

* * *

We decided to go to the beach. The sun and the sand would do me good, my caregiver advised. We used to laugh at the *trinkets* Singapore had. They had imported gadgets for everything. The Philippines made do with anything it could find—an unused umbrella, an abandoned stick. Such was the sand. Our brand of gadget, free for public use. We went as close to the seashore as my wheelchair allowed. The sand would provide a prickling, tickling sensation in my toes that would hopefully prod them to move.

There were a whole bunch of us who went. There were families seated on the sand around us. Some were barbecuing on their only day off, enjoying what precious little free things the tiny city-state offered them. People did extreme water sports in what seemed like a man-made lake, making me think of the abundance of clear blue waters and sandy shores we had at home.

They organized themselves to share the small lake. It amazed me with how much they did with what little they had.

It was a good day. There was no rain cloud in sight. The waves were inviting, the scenery expansive compared to the hospital views I had too much of. I just wished my family could see it. They had their backs turned to the waves. All gathered around my legs pouring sand solemnly and sullenly on my feet. It was not going to miraculously twitch while under their watch, but they continually poured sand on it anyway in silent but desperate expectation.

I wished for once I was not the centre of the universe. The world was passing them by, and they didn't notice. *How many days will they give up for me like that?* I looked at my mother. She had dropped all measure of vanity for me. Her hair was grey. She went into a store and bought all colours of a style of trousers as she could not be bothered to try various ones on. *Was I worth so many lives wasting away? How could I make the world not stop with me?*

* * *

It was to be my first non-touristy outing after the stroke. I had chosen a small bookstore to be my first foray into the outside world. I buried all my nervousness to attain a semblance of normalcy. I wanted to simply check out a bookstore.

It was in the outskirts of town, in what looked like a refitted old port building. We found ourselves surrounded by seas and container vans. It took less than a minute to scope the whole place out. The books lined up a wall from ceiling to floor, but that was it. There the celebrated photos plastered over the internet stopped.

We ordered everything on the menu in the small café tucked in the corner of the bookstore. There was rice topped with spam and wrapped with nori, sushi style, and that was it. There were three uninviting desserts that looked dry and old. We ordered them, nonetheless. We took our seats in one of the few tables, with me taking the foot of the table in my wheelchair.

We didn't know what else to do, so we visited the nearby near-empty museums. They were filled with modern young contraptions. Perhaps I was too old and unrefined to enjoy them, but we scoured the place anyway. We entered exhibits that seemed still in the making. In fact, they didn't let us pay for admission. We stopped at the adjacent art museum. They had an event going on, only no one was there. They had tables laid out for visitors to try some form of ancient charcoal art. We took our seats and tried to make some abstract black and white art. The place was absolutely deserted. Without anyone there, the press took photos of us as if we were intent on doing our masterpieces. That was as close as we came to being celebrities.

With still hours to kill before our ride picked us up, we decided to return to the museum housing the bookstore to try this computer-cum-vending machine churning out avatars. I picked a woman wearing shorts, a cap, and pearls in place of the simple non-frills mask holder I wore every day to rehab. It was my unofficial uniform. People had stuck printouts of their avatars on the wall of the museum. It turned out to be the museum's greatest hit. It seemed every living soul in the building lined up for it.

I am reminded of what St Hedwig said, 'All is narrow for me. I feel so vast.' It's amazing how much life there is to be led when we are not running, that there is time suddenly for savouring. What we're running to—do we really know? I remember roaming the streets of Rome finding the gelato store that supposedly sold the best gelato. I don't know how many times I passed the Trevi fountain to catch a glimpse of it. I don't know how much of Rome I saw. All I knew was that it was sundown, and I was in a foul mood when I stopped searching. What was I after? The chase? Who made it the best gelato anyway?

* * *

I sometimes forget my world has changed ever since the stroke or at least how the world treated me. FOMO (fear of missing out) and YOLO (you only live once) are really just taglines for those bustling with health that to lose it is some remote possibility. For those of us wheelchair-bound, FOMO and YOLO offer limited options.

But being handicapped does offer its perks too. One afternoon, we decided to catch *The LKY Musical*. What better way to learn about Singapore's founding father? We went to the venue two hours early, anticipating long lines. It was good that we came early because the show was apparently set to start one hour earlier than we originally thought. We had mixed up the times. We made it in the nick of time and heaved a sigh of relief. But it turned out we didn't have to worry because an usher pushed my wheelchair against the crowd, parting it as I went through it, shrieking in a shrill voice, 'Wheelchair!' The crowd gave way. I cowered in my seat and found myself apologetically at the beginning of the queue. It was a reality I was not used to, of things being made easy for me because I lost the sweepstakes where health was concerned.

You got to take some when you lose some. It is still startling for me to partake of a favour I was not born with. One weekend, we decided to see a talk by Ted Chiang who came to Singapore for a Writer's Festival. There was a book signing after his talk, but we were not harbouring hopes of actually meeting him. There were hundreds in attendance, and he had only an hour to sign books. Before his talk even officially ended, a crowd rushed down to the exit to line up for his book signing. That closed any chances for me as I still had to retrieve my parked wheelchair from where the people were exiting. We filed out slowly from the hall where he spoke. When an usher saw me, he offered to bring me straight to the start of the queue for the book signing. I barely had time to compose myself as the author strode out of the hall and planted himself before his adoring crowd and the press. He signed my books, *Exhalation* and *Stories of Your Life and Others*. I even got Kim who wheeled me to meet him. I felt self-conscious, as if all eyes were on me, as I met the author. I felt like living in sharp focus. I was dumbstruck like I'd never been before. The world does make it up to you when it can, and when it does, I just need to suck it up and make sure to keep my arms open.

51

My propensity to laugh has gotten me into social scrapes to my utter embarrassment. One day after rehab, we decided to get me some gym equipment. We went to this sports store full of all kinds of gym equipment, with a very loquacious owner manning the store. Out of the blue, the owner started showing us plans of a high-tech, fancy basketball court he was building in the Philippines. The earth would open up to reveal a hoop, magically, as if accompanied by heavenly music, whenever someone had the itch to play. He was so talkative, telling us things that we didn't need to hear that I burst out laughing.

It was a gargle of a laugh at first. I tried to hide it as if I was merely coughing, but it was no use. The laugh erupted from me like a pent-up volcano. I felt helpless to flee from my embarrassment. I was stuck in my chair, right in front of the owner trying my hardest to stare at the tumblers for sale to distract myself. In bouts of equanimity, I would keep a straight face, but it wouldn't last long. Soon enough, I would feel a laugh creeping in, with me trying to suppress it into deadly silent laughter until I couldn't contain it any longer, and the monstrous peals of laughter would wash over me. The owner, distracted, would look down at me, but seeing my wheelchair, would decide to forgive me. *Probably some nut in a wheelchair.* Trying to be respectful, the owner would try not to look at me, excluding me from the conversation and ignoring my peals of laughter. He would hold eye contact with everyone except me, as if I occupied some space vacuum that made me invisible. He was merciless; he didn't stop chatting. *Couldn't he see that he was torturing me?* My laughing fit was so terrible that Mimi wheeled me out of his store, excusing ourselves. Once out of his store, I let my laughter go, along with it any form of decorum. We moved away from his store, hoping that distance would forgive my laughter, but it only grew louder that I was practically bowled over 250 metres away. My mom, who was still helplessly stuck with the owner, later told me that she could hear my laughter inside the store.

52

Emily Dickinson wrote the poem, "'Hope" is the thing with Feathers'. 'Even in extremity, it never asked a crumb of me.' That was my favourite line in the poem. I often recounted it many times throughout my journey. Hope never robs you of what remains. It can only build you up. But faith is another beast altogether. It is fuel when you can't even see the end, when the tunnel is as dark as it is buried, when you can't figure out in what shape and form life will be back, if at all.

One afternoon, we went for my doctor's visit at his clinic in the hospital. We found ourselves off early in the afternoon. It was odd to have time in our own hands and to fill it how we wanted to. Our days were usually filled with therapy sessions and doctors' appointments. We decided to have early dinner at an al fresco restaurant by the bay. We ordered a whole chicken sitting atop a beer can surrounded by colourful and wholesome vegetables. We had it carved right in front of our eyes by a friendly Filipina server. The sky was blue and clear, the breeze friendly. We ordered corn dogs, sliders, and some sweet sugary drinks.

After dinner, we took a long stroll around the bay. We found ourselves in the middle of the tourist crowd as a new wax structure by Madame Tussaud's was about to be unveiled. No sooner had the red curtains unmasked the new structure did a crowd rush in with their cameras. Suddenly, in a flash, my vantage point was lost. People were towering above me as I sat in my wheelchair.

We wheeled away from the crowd. The lights across the bay started to come up as the sun slowly cast a warm orange glow on the horizon. I sat in my wheelchair and slowly navigated my way through tourists taking their photos along the bridge. We could see the Marina Bay Sands high and majestic across the bay. We could see the glistening crescent of the Bay's best offers. The skies quickly changed colours, as if its dark curtains were suddenly drawn. We crossed to the other side, taking the long scenic route to the Shoppes at Marina Bay mall, which had lighted Christmas trees suspended from the ceiling.

I looked around and felt as if I was unwrapping my present. There was only one way to go through the sights and sounds: slowly and in panoramic view. Suddenly, the light at the end of the tunnel was visible. I felt I could breathe wider. For the first time, I felt license to relax my shoulders and just enjoy the moment that was given back to me. Eight months ago, I would have been stuck in my bed in a dark room with my family crushed and sullen around me. But here we were. There was a light at the end of the tunnel after all. No one could grab away my present from me. It was like the world being re-gifted to me. It was glistening anew. It was about time the light showed itself to me, but I couldn't have hurried it either.

53

It happened when we were crossing the street. The air was cold around my neck. The people were bustling around with their paper bags, the Christmas air thick around them. Lively music blared through the public speakers and began greeting holiday travellers for the festive season. Lights streamed the sides of hotels to project holiday images. We were waiting to cross the street, the spaces filling beside us with hordes of people. *It was there when I felt it.* I looked to my right and left. People of all races, minding their own business, just wanting to cross the street. Some were clutching their holiday purchases; others were devouring ice cream sandwiches; still others came from the mosque at the corner of the street. For the first time in a long time, I felt the air free and careless to breathe, like I had the right to breathe the same air again as people did.

I had come out. Unbeknownst to me, I had trudged my way through the dark tunnel. I had surfaced from a hole I thought had no end, like one of those underground mazes in Vietnam, with tunnels leading into another until they made way to a large dining or even birthing room. It was amazing how much space could be found and made underground, but it was still underground. Stay underground long enough, and the dark becomes a friend. You forget that no matter how dark, it is still the dark. So, I didn't expect there to be a surfacing, the point when a swimmer breaks out of water and fills her lungs with air. The dark had been kind to me, but there was a world in the light to partake in. It was a world I knew too well, but it was also a world I knew the first time. The air was colder, purer. The music that played on the street was sweeter. Merry and bright—that was how the world received me.

54

Perhaps it was the world's way of telling me it was time to go home. I had been wanting to see my nurses before I left for home out of gratitude. I had a doctor's appointment in the hospital, so I stepped in the hallowed halls of the Singapore hospital that took me under its wing for six weeks. Familiar smells and scenes greeted me. I know a hospital is supposed to scare you, but I looked at mine with particular familiarity and fondness. I would always find my way around that hospital.

While waiting for the lift, a familiar face stood across me waiting to go up too. It was Zenaida, my ICU nurse who took it upon herself to take care of me like I was family even if I wasn't. Even if she knew me just on the day, half conscious. Her hair was wet, as if she just rushed to work. She had a coffee hanging on her hand and was still in plain clothes. 'Zenaida,' I muttered. She looked at me unsurely. It was all I could do not to hug her. She was an angel in disguise.

Then I was on my way to rehab when the elevator doors opened and in came two veteran nurses from the neurology ward, Halina and KK. They were nursing a sprain and planned to amble their way to the clinic across rehab. What were the odds? If the universe was telling me something, it was spelling it out for me now. I was homeward bound, and I had to come to grips with it.

55

The spirit of trauma is not a sharp cutting pain that wants to eat you alive. At least it was not for me. It was a dull, unknowing pain that ate at me. I didn't want to return. I wanted to move forward, but I guess some things you have to return to in order to move forward. Otherwise, it would just be a turning back.

I planned my remaining time in Singapore carefully. I had made new friends. I had made a new life. There was Henry with his crutches. There were tubes connected to his arm to course through his antibiotics. Even so, he lived alone and thought he was not sick, merely unfortunate. He swam with his one good leg. He had his meals at this fancy Chinese restaurant. He was such a preferred guest that they delivered food to his home when he needed it. I almost choked on my dinner when he casually mentioned his family owned a golf course. I didn't know of any individual who owned a golf course. He always wore a white tee and blue jeans. We figured he was some crazy rich Asian cum venture capitalist.

Henry was like family in our apartment. We kept track when he was to have his next surgery and shopped fruits for him. He started having English lessons with Kim in the garden. We made home-cooked meals for him. We ate dim sum together. We think he paid for my harrowing acupuncture sessions because they didn't cost a cent. Imagine getting anything for free in Singapore. He came twice with us to the sessions just to translate for us. It was an unexpected kindness from a stranger that is hard to trust these days. But here he was, our angel in disguise.

There was also this incredibly warm dad, Mickael, whom we always rubbed shoulders with in the elevator. He would, while flustered, always have time for his children. He would sit in a remote meeting one second, then play ball with his daughters in the next. His wife and son were arriving from their Korean vacation the next day, so he was celebrating his last night alone with his daughters with Pepsi. His twin daughters, Giulia and Emma, looked like they were about to attend a party by invitation only, like a couple of teenagers. The mom, Stefanie, and the older brother, James, about seven, had gorgeous curly brown hair. The kids loved the water. We almost always spotted them at the pool without fail. I practiced walking to a nearby mall to get the kids cookies as an errand for myself. They were moving out of the apartment, so we cooked a special dish from home for them to taste—adobo with a twist. Here was a family diving headlong into Asia. They needed a proper introduction.

They invited us to their new home shortly before we left. They served a French breakfast of bread, jam, and eggs. We brought toys for the kids supposedly for their first Christmas in Singapore, but the gifts didn't stay wrapped for too long. We had a nice, leisurely breakfast, two families who couldn't possibly have met without fate intervening. It was a good Sunday.

Then there was Sajeda from London whose husband, Naveed, was recently transferred to work in Singapore. We always saw her everywhere around the apartment. Finally, she broke the silence and inquired about me in the elevator. Her mom had a stroke too and she assumed I, by the way I was ambling around, had one too. She was the friendliest person I met at the apartment. She gave me a book, *The Secret*, a book she constantly carried with her, in case someone needed it. She rang at our apartment's door several times to visit with us. It was a serviced apartment that we were staying at, but her warmth gave us a home.

Then there was Heather, a sprightly, well-dressed thin woman who was forever collecting steps to reach ten thousand. She would walk to-and-fro, covering the area of the garden with resolve in her steps while conducting her social life through her phone in her hands. She befriended everyone in the building. She knew all the stroke victims soaking some sun in the garden. She barely spoke English, but she didn't let that stop her. She gathered names of doctors and wrote them on tiny slips of paper to give to anyone who needed it per chance. She wasn't that lucky herself. She was recovering from breast cancer. One day, she made us some mango sticky rice with caramel. She had brought the ingredients from Indonesia. On a bright sunny afternoon, we ate her homemade sticky rice, going out on a limb by taking our masks off, our deficits trailing by.

Many months later, we saw Heather again when she returned for her regular check-up in Singapore. She was billeted in another hotel, but she still messaged to see us. She was coming from the hospital after her blood extractions, trudging a carry-on filled with goodies from Indonesia. We met her while waiting for our turn to see Dr Lee in his clinic. We chatted with her broken English and our barely-there Mandarin, care of Duolingo. How many would care to see a friend across the seas that she's shared sticky rice with only once? I guess we broke bread that one time.

We knew everybody, every long staying guest that came and went. We were at the apartment for six months. It had become our sprawling grounds. The bell captain, Devandran, welcomed my family to our soon-to-be apartment building when they were apartment hunting. He and his aides saw us in every taxi ride and waved us goodbye until we were out the driveway like they knew us intimately. He even invited us to his place to spend Diwali. Such overreaching kindness. It was hard to say goodbye to it all.

56

The time finally came to say goodbye. It was inevitable. I had to wrap up our time in Singapore. It had its time. First, there were my 'classmates' to say goodbye to, people I saw almost every day in rehab. They were as much a fixture there as I was. They were a picture of struggle and hard work. If their input matched that of their output, they would have long been distance runners.

Second, there were my therapists. I got the luck of the draw. To actually like my therapists when I saw them twice a day for more than six months was more than I could ask for. I actually looked forward to rehab.

Third, there was the place of my recovery, Singapore. I laughingly told my friends that before the stroke, I had wanted to live long-term in a first world country, just to know how it felt like. I got my wish. Living eight months in Singapore before the stroke would have been unthinkable. There would have been too much to leave behind. Living in a new place undoubtedly spurred my recovery. Everything piqued my interest. I felt a joyous dawning every time I realized how a Singlish phrase came to be used. *It was a direct translation of Chinese! You see how, can or not?* The phrases suddenly made sense to me. It spoke of their culture and their people. Singapore fed the learner in me. I couldn't turn off because there were so many new things to learn. I tasted Peranakan food; I wheeled in their local markets; I hobbled through their heritage sites; I traipsed through their probably uncelebrated boardwalks. I was like an incapacitated traveller, but a traveller, nonetheless.

To be honest, it was in a sense the most carefree vacation I've had in years.

Finally, there was my primary doctor. I loved visiting his clinic for my monthly visits. We always had silly quips and musings for each other. He had become a fast friend. I would always credit my speedy recovery to his ability to see past my sickness. He didn't let me drown in the severity of my condition, medical facts that apparently matter least when you're impaired. He would have been stating the obvious, and I didn't need any of that. Instead, he created opportunities for laughter. Every time I visited him, I always wrote him a letter to accompany a little gift, often of an inside joke we shared. On one last visit before we went home, probably sensing my trepidation at leaving, he brandished a handwritten letter. I could hardly contain my tears. What a fitting farewell.

I relished the time shortly after my discharge when I did not fear death. I knew with a definitiveness that when it was your time to go that it was your time to go. There was no negotiating it. When it wasn't your time, no matter the suffering, it wasn't your time. You're going to get through it. It was an extremely liberating feeling. Neither death nor life had a grip on me. Because I wasn't yet particularly attached to life, I felt I wasn't giving up much upon death. We cling so much to life only to waste it. I thought from when I started to lose my life. Clearly, I lost it much earlier than the stroke. The stroke only helped me to find it back.

The suffering was so great that I was sure a great joy was coming. It was a feeling so sure that I was excited about the rejoicing in the thick of my sorrow. What would I give to have that sureness in everyday life? There is a time to sow and a time to reap. It was finally time to be expectant.

Part 4

57

I knew I had landed in the Philippines when the supposed automatic door of the handicapped comfort room would not close. I was weary to traverse a familiar place as an invalid. While I was not ashamed about my plight, I dreaded the questions that I expected were headed my way.

It was not the first time I had stepped into our airport, but it was my first time wheelchair-bound. In many ways, the airport experience was a breeze. I was given privilege in queues, to board first, to alight last. It was like being on fast track in Disney World.

We made our way out of the airport and boarded our car. The traffic jam met us like a force to reckon with. It took us hours to get to our relatively nearby home, passing by dirty highways, faulty traffic lights, and a myriad of tiny colourful stores with unique names only a Filipino can have. It was a sight of people fending for themselves. The government seemed invisible, more a liability than a safety net. It was a sight to get used to, yet it was a sight I was used to. I once was very proud of it.

It seemed the Philippines had only grown poorer the time that we were away, or we had only grown accustomed to first-world living the past eight months. Either way, this was my home, my home that had so desperately failed me. I had to come to terms with that. My doctor once told me that there was this teacher who got a stroke. When she returned to her old teacher's chair, she broke down as if on cue. I was afraid of that. I didn't know what power the past and my home had on me. But here I was facing the inevitable. Not to go home would have been avoidance. I would be all patched up yet with a gaping hole inside. I didn't want that. Handicapped as I was, I wanted to be completely whole.

58

Everything in the Philippines was unpredictable. We didn't opt to go to the rehabilitation centres because we would spend the whole day on the road because of the traffic jams. We opted for home rehabilitation instead. We started the third day we got home. We set up a home gym in the living room with the implements we got from Singapore.

My physical therapist, Luis, was a soft-spoken guy who was previously a bodybuilder. I thought it was difficult to find a physical therapist in Cebu. I could not imagine anyone better than Siva, but he had his own charm. Slowly, I found myself training as an athlete. We built on what Siva built. He focused on rebuilding my strength.

He badly wanted me to activate my command centre. Aggressive manual therapy, he called it. I struggled with enormous effort and with bated breath to produce the littlest movement. I was wrestling with my own body. I wanted to activate one set of muscles, but another would overpower it. I seemed to have nursed a combatant against me inside my own body. I couldn't get my muscles to talk to each other even if I wanted to. It was like they were controlled by two separate brains. I did sit-to-stands, sumo squats, and mini lunges until my muscles were sore. Standing for normals seemed easy enough, but standing, to me, felt like straightening an iron rod planted in my back. Moving my legs felt like stretching a taut rubber band.

Stretching my arms felt like ungluing concrete. Despite our repetitious routines, he kept things light. I called him Coach.

I was lucky with my occupational therapist. She was an anchor I needed in the Philippines. Cebu threw off all reliable routines, a major thing that saved my life in Singapore. It is difficult to imagine that I was used to this very fluid life before the stroke that required negotiation at every turn, but Pria was a constant upon going home. She gave me the reliability I needed.

If I had any pride left, occupational therapy would have been an insult to my person. We made a Valentine's Day card out of red scrap paper which I picked up with my gnarly fingers to stick to a printed outline of a heart on my card. We dipped cotton buds in poster paint and dotted them on pre-printed dots across a sheet of paper. The exercise made me move my arms and fingers across all directions lightly and functionally. It reminded me very strongly of the kind of art I did in kindergarten. Good thing I never read anything more into what I was doing.

No matter how we tried to liven up therapy sessions, we could only do so much. In truth, the Philippines, I found, was drab. There was nowhere to go save for the ultra-big hotels and supermarkets. I could go nowhere. Resources and options for the handicapped were severely limited. Good luck finding continuous paved sidewalks to wheel on.

One day, I finally agreed to venture out the confines of my home. I didn't know what drew more eyes, being in a wheelchair or being off it and hobbling helplessly. It was my first time to actually walk into a restaurant after the stroke. I limped, relying heavily on family to walk me through the aisles. I could feel the eyes of those sitting al fresco on me. I could almost make out the expressions on their faces without looking at them. It was a painfully long walk, but at least I was shorn of that self-consciousness nagging nastily at normal people when there is nothing wrong with them, when no one is staring at them. Now everyone was staring at me, but I wasn't self-conscious. They were staring at my disability, not at myself. I felt a relief wash over me as I finally divorced myself from my disability.

I was forced to make use of my time like I never had before. I decided to 'befriend' my therapist's other patients. We were in the same boat after all. There was a grandmother, Elizabeth, who loved to read. I never met her, but I heard *about* her. I sent her poetry books through Coach, she sent me desserts made uniquely of birdseed in return. I felt like the protagonist in *The Guernsey Literary and Potato Peel Pie Society*. I ordered a McDonald's breakfast every Saturday so I could look forward to something every week. I had my caffeine fix every weekend. I frequented this homey café which I loved because of its wide walkways and squeaky-clean washroom. *I could actually fit my wheelchair in the washroom!* I learned to make little things celebratory.

It turned out what my country lacked in facilities, it doubled down on in human resource. There was a lot more empathy than in Singapore. I guess that was how it was in a country accustomed to hardship and loss. The wait staff and the guards at the café knew me already. They would remark about my progress every time I visited. I tried not to hate my city. I tried to think like it didn't owe me anything. For sure, I loved it considerably less, but it didn't fail me. I came to terms with it just being it. I lived in a third-world country, plain and simple.

59

I was obsessed with Ina Garten. She helped me fill my days. I curated our meals for lunch and dinner and made do with ingredients we had in the pantry. I started with simple dishes until I advanced to more experimental ones. My newfound obsession with food brought me out of the house. I scoured supermarket aisles like a kid let loose in a candy store. Suddenly produce seemed a lot more exciting. I drew inspiration from what I saw in the aisles. I got myself an Instant Pot and had jolly good fun with it. Seldom would you find the kitchen without the Instant Pot or the oven churning something. I finished watching almost all of Ina's cooking videos on YouTube and added a few unhelpful kilos to my stature.

I understand that there is nothing special about loving cooking. But I don't know how my present state of life would be without it. How different would it be? Cooking gave me a routine in this new unpredictable environment. As sure as the sun would rise in the morning and set in the evening, my stomach would ask for lunch and dinner. Someday I would thank cooking for its earnest efforts in my recovery.

60

I reopened my old drawers. It was bound to happen sooner or later. I couldn't ignore it any longer if I wanted to move on with my life. It was like unearthing relics that seemed like mine, but were too detailed and advanced. If I was living life in broad strokes now, I was then living in the minutiae.

I looked at memos I wrote to the government. Some involved math that I should not have had business with. I was trying to break down a calculation for the department that should have understood it most in the first place. I remember my dealings with it being a steep uphill climb, trying to make the officers apply the law on matters that looked slightly different than what they're used to. The exercise was an example of the Philippines' brand of making mountains out of molehills. I struggled to understand what I wrote. It was not because I couldn't understand the work but because I was rusty. I was painfully aware that I was one of the few who could still deal with complex thoughts. I was and could still be a lawyer.

I remember in my early days in rehab, there was this perfectly normal-looking guy climbing up a fake staircase. The therapist introduced him as a lawyer. It was funny—lawyers still being highly looked up to in an arena that would have plainly spelled out what their work is about. The place was littered with lawyers. The guy asked from what firm I came from, a common question between lawyers. Later, I found out that he could no longer practice law. Sure, he could climb stairs and make polite small talk, but he couldn't make a pleading or face a judge. He could not deal with more complex thought. I didn't know why my severing arteries decided to stop just before claiming my higher mental faculties. I wondered what it was like to make small talk about a profession I couldn't go back to. My past would be a constant slap in the face.

I leafed through all my files, intricate dealings with the government that were just not worth it. If the face of the government didn't know its own law, good luck convincing them about it. I fought tooth and nail for what was legally expected in the simplest of circumstance. In the end, my life was composed of arguments just haunting me from the page. I looked at the pages that revealed my life, the intensity of it. It was just one strand of my life. I remember thinking to myself shortly before the stroke that I was wearing too many hats. *What caused my stroke?* Despite people wanting me to go forward, I couldn't help but occasionally look back to that question. When the dust settled, I needed an answer. I couldn't wrap my head around the fact that my defective artery was just inborn.

61

My shelves of books stared at me. I had owned a budding online bookstore, Blithe Books, just before I had the stroke. Now, I had almost a year's worth of unsold books just staring at me. Some of them had lost their timing, their 'coming out' because I was sick. I was inundated with yellowing books. The books were the backdrop of my life as I did my therapy every day, as if kindling me back to life.

I started tinkering with them, picking out and making collections out of them. When I was done with a newly created collection, I would begin with what I thought was a harmless another. But the world creeps in innocuously like that. *How fast did I voluntarily give up my newfound freedom with the noise of the world?* To think Blithe work was work that I loved. How much more did I squeeze myself doing things I detested to allow for the seeming folly of Blithe? The world turns something beautiful into something toxic if we let it. We fill our lives unknowingly until we are too caught to get out. By the time I retreated, I had redone inventory, prepared for my reopening, formed a non-profit, and thought to hire lawyers to make local hospitals become stroke-ready at the threat of litigation. I had almost deceived myself into thinking that I could do anything, but I couldn't. No matter my wilfulness, I knew that with certainty now. I couldn't even save myself. I had to do things differently.

* * *

Getting back to life was a novel challenge. I got to dangle my feet in the water before I immersed myself in it. I got to decide when I was ready. But does that time ever come? Is there ever a time when we unwrap ourselves as a brand-new toy in a box? I was as brand new as I ever was going to be.

We decided to open the bookstore one Saturday on Instagram. All my tinkering with the books was bound to culminate in the reopening somehow, no matter how crippled our operations were. I didn't work with the feverish intensity that possessed me before, taking a step forward before I fully left one. I still approached my business with a fiery passion, but I was set free somehow. I didn't need to chase things. I had nothing to prove, no one to please. If you liked me, it was because you liked what I put out. It was liberating to feel that way. Unwittingly, I had lived on the world's terms before.

We opened slowly but surely. Our opening was not with a bang but a more tamed foray into bookstagram. We had closed for almost a year, but it was heartwarming how we never left our old customers' reverie. Our oldest customers welcomed us right back, as if life never happened in between. They sent me personal messages. I even found our old customer who gave me a Neruda recording in the ICU. I listened to it every day. I realized we forged lasting relationships in our short stint as an independent bookstore. Our customers posted videos of their unboxing, tagging us as they happily received their books. It was a wave we happily rode on. I struggled to reply to messages with my left hand only. I typed at a snail's pace. I took photographs of the books while I could hardly stand and balance (to my phone screen's demise because it broke). But life was sweet. It was like we lived the last year in a vacuum. We were unaware what the people were reading, where they posted about it, and generally the local beat. TikTok invited us to be part of Booktok, and I was ignorant of both. But awkwardly, we had one step back in the door. Crippled or not, we were back.

We resurrected our fledgling subscription program, Blithely, one Saturday. What a joy that people seemed to be almost nostalgic about it and wanted to resubscribe. We put our website back up. We started a reading club, The Tortoise and the Hare—a new project. We had lost our momentum at our first run, but Blithe Books came back with a maturity I would not trade.

I can't measure what my tiny bookshop did for me in my recovery. It kept for me the last strands of adulthood that had so easily left me. No one knew how exactly I left the bookshop when I got the stroke but me. No one knew how to dispose of a thousand books in inventory but me. My passion ran deep in Blithe Books' veins. The bookstore gave me a sense of responsibility to wake up every morning because I still had something other than for myself to do. It was an outlet for me to go beyond myself when everything else was centred on me.

* * *

Back in Singapore, the weekend after my discharge, finding I could do nothing, I got myself a tablet and downloaded a year's worth of Audible. If I couldn't read well with my eyes, at least I could listen to my books. Somehow though, I couldn't give up on reading that easily. I wheeled myself to a Kinokuniya across the street and picked up a copy of *Letter to my Younger Self* presented by The Big Issue. It was a book of short essays. It was good for non-committal, nonchalant reading. In idle periods, I would slowly go through an essay, never really expecting to finish the book. When I had read up to three quarters of the book, it suddenly dawned on me that I could finish the book. My eyesight had straightened itself out enough for me to read the lines more clearly. I planted myself in the garden and decided to dedicate an hour to just reading.

It turned out to more than just save my eyes. While stuck in my wheelchair, the books provided a playground for my mind that it never became idle. It made my otherwise monotonous days unpredictable. It made me forget about the dreary position I was in. *Let your mind roam free.* That used to be my tagline in the bookshop. It could not have been more useful to me then. After the book on essays, I casually read *Bird by Bird* by Anne Lamott, *Tattoos on the Heart* and *The Whole Language* by Gregory Boyle, *Finding Freedom in the Lost Kitchen* by Erin French, and *The Lost Continent* by Bill Bryson, with an enthusiasm of a kid who had just discovered reading. I rooted for French as she built the Lost Kitchen (which was concurrently the namesake of a show I was hooked on in Magnolia network), laughed at Fr Boyle's anecdotes, and travelled with Bryson as he drove himself through small town America. I will always be grateful for their distraction.

I gave my therapists new books most every month, whether they seemed interested in reading or not. I also gave my 'classmates' random books until rehab caught a reading bug. My therapists started giving me books of their interest. We joked about starting a book club together. I finally got the cue to stop giving out unsolicited books when Siva said he was staring at a tableful of unread books when we got to the third month of therapy.

I remember, in my childhood, my father, upon travelling to Manila, would call us who were back at home and personally read to us the titles of the books that were available over the phone. There was a dearth of bookstores where we were at. Having access to a Manila bookstore was joyous and special. We would stock up on titles for the summer. We have come a long way it seems, the books and I.

62

I learned a lot about my brain while it was under repair. I learned how it learned, what to expect from it, when to expect from it. It was like watching a football match in slow motion. I got the play by play for all the scenes. It was like the most basic chunky cogs of my brain were working hard to get the most basic of plays down.

I was getting reacquainted with my brain in a way few people had the chance to. It was scary, but there was no way to experience it but through it. How was it like when you first swallowed? How did it feel when you first stood upright keeping your balance? I could feel my core muscles tugging, pulling, maintaining a centre to keep me on air. I was like a tree trunk on roller blades. I remember going under the water in a swimming pool and realizing too late that my nose and my throat had forgotten to coordinate to allow me to do just that. I coughed up water like a child learning to swim for the first time.

No matter how difficult the first try was, I knew my brain ultimately learned. It wasn't taking its sweet time either. It was trying its damn hardest to keep me functioning. Every movement required a mental rehearsal, like a parent handholding a child at every milestone. *Mind your thumb. Square your hip. Make sure your feet are flat on the ground before standing.* Just as much as it let me down, my brain built myself up. It was a thrill to see I was getting better. I was jumping from miracle to miracle. I gained back my head control. I noticed that as the nurses tried to carry my weight by a lifter, I could help lessen the weight by carrying my own head, which was pretty heavy. I recovered my eyesight, speech, and ability to swallow. My rectal and bladder muscles started working. The day my catheter was removed was a happy day—I no longer had to lug around a bag of my pee to therapy. I didn't plateau. My walking improved day by day. I was painfully aware that I was improving significantly faster than others, my case having been severe. I admired the patience my occupational therapist had to catch a minute advancement of my progress every day. Ten to twenty to thirty degrees, my arms opened toward its side. After a few tries of my fingers barely grasping a block, it could now manage to clumsily do so. I began to grip an oversized spoon and fork. Like a child, I would haphazardly spoon food to my mouth like a downed jet spiralling down. I would meet the spoonful with my mouth, my head compensating for the lack of control in my arm. My therapist said there was no small wins in this business. The chance of being conscious at every learning turn was priceless.

* * *

Recovering from a stroke was like watching my brain reboot. You know how when you painfully watch your computer reboot little by little? It's like that. You think you have completely grasped a situation until your brain reaches another milestone and your brain accommodates more, and you find that something you thought you completely understood before, you never really wrapped your head around until now.

'Hip forward,' was what the therapists always said, since what seems like time immemorial. I was boggled by how to do it, but I just thrusted my way around in a way I thought was right. One day, while standing for a long time redecorating our house, it dawned on me where my hip was. It was an awareness of this huge chunk of bone in my body, this massive fulcrum that held my weight. Keeping it in the centre spelt the difference between falling and standing. It was a hallelujah moment for me. It was like a dozen instructions held in abeyance in mid-air finally came to a full meaning for me. I was not merely following a manual. I had earned the capacity of an engineer for my own body.

Just as quickly as it snuck up on me, the awareness was quickly absorbed by my body. It disappeared. Such was the quandary. I thought I held my brain, but my body had a brain of its own. If you were normal, you wouldn't need to know where your hip was. It held its function so well that you just knew it as part of yourself. But apparently it was not as intuitive for a halfwit like me. It was a learned thing. The day I learned it, I felt like I advanced in years. That must be how a baby grows. Except a baby has all his or her childhood years to grow up awkwardly. I have nary the time.

When I was in rehab, my therapists kept pulling and tugging at my arm. I saw it go up and down, in and out, but I couldn't feel it deliberately moving. I thought they were tricking me. 'Is it me moving?' I would muse. I didn't feel the connection. I gave the order, but the transmission lines were badly burnt. Still, my therapists were patient with me. They worked with mere potentiality, and it didn't harrow them.

The thing about being a halfwit is that I knew that if I continually learned, I could grow into a full wit. The process was painfully long, and it was painful to be in it, but while I could not be certain about the destination, I could be certain about the process. There was something liberating about knowing your increments can add up to something. My brain, I found, was suddenly my biggest ally while it was healing itself. It must be true what they say, you start becoming old when you stop learning.

I don't know how my recovery would have gone if I had let myself plunge myself into the darkness before everything started. How lonely that place must be. It must be enveloping, my incapacity. It must be a large black lagoon to swim circles in.

63

One day, I was riding in the car, my face pressed to the window. We were on our way back from a seaside town in an attempt to catch the shore. We found out too late that there was no access for the handicapped, and we were forced to admire the sea from afar. As we were rolling slowly down the street adjacent to the sea, I saw him. He was ambling down an undone cement bridge. He had a limp on his right. He appeared to be dragging the right side of his body along with him. He strode nonchalantly on the road leading with his left. He stopped by a friend, sitting on the bridge for a chat. *So that is how a stroke looked on the outside.* It was like looking through a mirror. I didn't need to ask him. I knew what he had. I knew it so intimately. So that is how it must have gone by if I was not this privileged lady sent to rehab in Singapore. If I had not died nor been brought to Singapore, I would have found a way to live my life. I would have learned to live with my sickness, as if it were the shirt on my back. My friends remained the same. The sea remained the same. I had to find the lemons that remained in me to make my lemonade.

64

I once asked my mother if the standards now that I was handicapped were different. I felt I could do no wrong whereas before my clumsiness easily disappointed and irked my loved ones. She assured me that they weren't different. They're not, but they were. Well-meaning, my caregiver would swoop in with a towel to wipe off my sweat and place it underneath my shirt, like I was a ten-year-old in a playground, as I would chat with my therapists in a gym full of grown people. I would transfer to my commode half-naked, somehow it not occurring to her to close the blinds because who could care less? The standards are not different, but they were. We lost a lot more than our bodies.

65

It was like a Christmas gift waiting to be opened. The day had finally come when we were to return to Singapore for a follow-up check-up. I dressed in a long-sleeved shirt and sweatpants for my trip. The shirt was lavender and the pants a pale pink, colours I would not have chosen for myself before the stroke. Heck, I would have relegated a lavender and pink colour combination to the bygone years of childhood, but being sick wiped out all notions of what was for a child and what was for an adult.

Being in a wheelchair at the airport was a little like being a nun in a habit. Everyone felt comfortable saying hi to me even if I didn't know them. I received the stares, the looks, and the smiles as I was strolled in. People were extra nice and helpful to me. I half-wished everyone saw what I saw—how the world felt a few feet shorter. It was a new playing field I was not familiar with. What were the rules on this side of the world? I was sure it was not only honey and roses as in the airport. The world can be sweet and savage at the same time.

The wheelchair brought me to the mouth of the plane, whereupon I hobbled to my seat. It was not a special seat at the front of the plane. It was a seat like anybody else's. I was the last one to board the plane. I felt all eyes on me. I felt every second fly by until I got to my seat. I plopped on my seat with satisfaction. I had always fancied that feeling of bringing a book with me up in the plane and reading it in the still of mid-air. As a lawyer, many times had I hopped on a plane, donning a power outfit and carrying a book in my purse, with hardly the time to actually read a page or two. I was living the life mid-air.

Part 5

66

I stared at the images that flew by me in my taxi's window in Singapore, as if staring hard enough would commit them to memory. Here I was, back in a place that was so forgiving to me. I took in the sight of the greenery, and the tall buildings, and the paved roads, and the clean air that greeted me. I read once that people make the mistake of bringing their entire lives in a new place, mistakenly hoping that the new place would inject something fresh into their lives. I wasn't entirely new, but the stroke did give me a good scrubbing that led me to see the city with fresh eyes.

We settled in our new apartment without issue. Riding a taxi to rehab, I saw a *Frozen* musical ad sprawled on the sides of a taxi. It was not exactly something I wanted to see, but I knew I wanted to watch a musical. Chances at catching one in the Philippines were slim.

So right then and there, we decided to watch *Frozen* that evening. We took a cab to Marina Bay Sands to see the spectacle. Kim almost laughed her heart out when she saw the throng of 'people' dressed to watch the musical. They were clad in yards of blue and white taffeta with their hair in braids and generally under four feet tall. We found ourselves inching slowly towards the theatre's entrance amidst kids. Everything was blue. The popcorn was sprinkled with blue glittering powder. The refreshments were bubble gum in flavour. The delectable treats all bore the shade of the heroine, Elsa. The show turned out to be more than we expected it to be. Perhaps it was the crowd. They joined in song uninhibitedly at every popular refrain. The theatre would fill with the joyful and angelic voices of babes. Every time the jovial snowman would appear, the crowd would burst into giggles and laughter. Their laugh was more entertaining than the scene playing out in front of me. It was whole, as if nothing plagued them at the back of their minds. It was cheaply given, wholesome and unabashed. It didn't take long to tickle them gleefully. My mom and Kim stood up in standing ovation as the cast came out before the final curtain. Clouds of silver and blue dust rained from the sky as the crowd shrieked in delight. People started shoving silver dust in the air.

I watched the scene from my wheelchair at the last row of the theatre. I couldn't help thinking I had just endured the worst of my predicament. It was the first real time my mom, sister, and I got a breather. It was the first time we got to sit down and just enjoy the show. It was only fitting that a bunch of kids greeted us back to life. No other calculated adult moment could have reintroduced us to and encapsulated life for us as those kids. I felt happy and relieved for Kim and my mom. My pain was their pain. It permitted no holiday. It was love that admitted only black or white. It couldn't accept grey.

We spent the rest of the night walking along the bay enjoying the cool air around us, not minding the time. Kim took touristy photos. It was a precious gift—the all-elusive time deciding to spend a few lackadaisical moments in life. I am reminded of what my doctor said in one of my visits to him. He who laughs last laughs best.

67

I accompanied my aunt who came with us to Singapore to see Dr Wee, the covering neurologist who first received me in Singapore. I wanted to show him my progress, that I could now limp and amble towards his clinic. Boy, did I make a huge blunder. When the kind neurologist asked her what she was feeling, she began enumerating every disease since time immemorial. She had a frozen shoulder and had contracted meningitis about twenty-five years ago. When asked when she last had a headache, she answered that her headaches usually occurred every day at 11 p.m., which led the doctor to deduce that she was probably sleepy at that hour. She would slip blissfully into bouts of nothingness too, expecting her son who accompanied us and me to answer for her, except that we didn't, and there would be an air of silence hanging over us. I would burst into unforgiving laughter in these pockets of solemn silence. I pitied my cousin. He tried to keep me at bay, answer for his mom, and inject some comedy in the atmosphere to excuse our comedic act. I tried desperately to recover any professionalism left in me. I would achieve lucid intervals about a minute long when I would stare listlessly at a potted plant like a deranged patient. Dr Wee couldn't help it. Finally, he asked, 'What's so funny?' I apologized for my random fits of laughter. Let's call a spade a spade. It was either that or irrepressible sobbing. I answered that my cousin was really a jokester, but I was responsible for my embarrassing fit. He nodded understandably like a neurologist only could. 'Keep her happy,' he mused. Then to my aunt, who had gone as far as her urinary tract infection at some unknown time, he said sombrely, 'Let's stick to the brain.'

68

The week before I was to come to Singapore, Jack, a friend from rehab messaged Kim. He was asking about how I was doing at home. He had always been one of the more 'normal' guys in rehab. Except for a small and intermittent shake, you could hardly tell he was sick. He was a litigation lawyer. He was always professional, friendly, and independent. He walked himself in and out of rehab. That was a big thing.

So, on my first visit back in rehab, I asked about my classmates. Some had returned to Indonesia. Others had graduated. Others had gone to seek 'greener' pastures in another rehabilitation centre. But Jack—we didn't hear of him. One day later, we received word that Jack was confined in the hospital and that he could no longer move. I was aghast. *That nimble Jack that strode almost effortlessly in rehab.*

I was suddenly made aware of how close I had come to desolation and how close I come to it every day. There is a shock that comes at first. *How could this previously completely mobile person in one instant be this block of stone?* I guess that must be how my family felt when they looked at me in the early days. They must have seen, protested, and vehemently objected to my fading future.

What would have become of me if my brainstem tore a centimetre more? Just a centimetre more? My life would have been vastly different. *Would I have been able to carry the torch they do every day? For how long? What if I didn't have the insurance money to save myself?* Why did God not just finish the job in the most severe of cases?

Being gone seemed an easier pill to swallow than having a highly functioning cognitive brain trapped in an immobile body that can't swallow or talk.

The patients in rehab had families at home waiting for them. What was a wife, newly married, at the cusp of life with a myriad expectations, to do for a lifetime with an infirm husband at her side? What was the husband to do? To want to continue to live bore a price of its own.

I couldn't help thinking the worst about people who disappeared in rehab. *Why did they stop coming? Did anything worse happen to them? How do I know I won't have a stroke again?* I learned that something bad is as close to you as something good. Something that will knock our socks off is just lurking around the corner. Sadly, it has not been the invincibility of life that has taught me to live but its frailty.

69

I wonder when I 'regressed' into a child. By no accounts do I think being childlike a 'regression', but you know what I mean. I was still an adult in the ICU. I was still an adult in the hospital in Singapore. There were nurses and medical staff to answer to. My illness was new. I had to adjust to a lot of changes. But then discharge came, and I was left in the charge of my family all day. I couldn't do anything in the early days, so I was dependent on them for absolutely everything. They bathed me; they dressed me. I got used to that routine of dependence, and I guess whether I liked it or not, it had a subconscious effect on my psyche. Slowly, I found myself acting more and more child-like, with mannerisms and facial expressions like that of a child. I told my mother that if I did the things I did now before the stroke (like deciding not to take part in an adult conversation at the dinner table), I would have been banished from my household. My illness gave me license not to care about things. With less and less things on my plate, I became more carefree. I did not carry a wallet (that luxury I had in Singapore of just flashing a watch to pay for goods was taken from me in the Philippines). I hardly went out. I did not drive. I was a stark contrast to my previously able self. I yawned like a baby. My arms and fingers curled and clawed involuntarily exactly like a baby's. My dad talked to me in an artificially upbeat voice. I had not been talked to like that since I was a toddler. My environment was nurturing me to be like a child. In my diminished fitness, I relieved myself of the responsibilities of an adult.

Part 6

70

I didn't know what I was gunning for at that date. I didn't know why I was marking it either. It was hard to believe that it had been almost a year since the incident that obtrusively interrupted and radically changed my life. When I recently had the stroke, the question that rang the loudest in my mind was, *For how long?* A year to recover seemed almost unbearable and unacceptable. And yet, here we were now. This was how the almost one-year mark looked, and I had made it triumphantly.

For my first-year anniversary back in the Philippines, I decided to go to the beach. Just nature unhampered and unadulterated. Broad and vast and peaceful. Maybe that's what I was supposed to be. I once heard that people who watch the sunrise have increased well-being. For some reason the thought stuck to me. I wanted to do something vastly different from what I was doing a year ago. I decided to go to the tip of my island to watch the sunrise. Four hours away through the mountains with no idea where to go pee—it would be my first long road trip away from home.

71

I reached a beach resort at the tip of our island, set on catching what I came for. I don't think I've woken up at 5.30 a.m. since reviewing for the bar exam. I guess it spoke about my drastic shift in life views since then. I ambled in the dark until I reached my wheelchair in the terrace of the room we were staying in. Hurriedly, Kim and I walked to the edge of the shore to catch the sunrise. The sun hid behind murky clouds. Our first sunrise was a disappointment.

We then headed to the beach, which seemed like a vast expanse of rice paddies after the tides had retreated. We settled ourselves where the tides met the sand. I unfolded a plastic stool and dangled my feet in the foamy water.

There was the lifeguard Don-Don and the security guard, Rivera, keeping a close eye on us. With the way I was walking, it was impossible not to draw stares. Curious, they asked about me. Then, they started talking. My reverie was opened to a treasure trove of indigenous practices the province held for stroke. It would be a common provincial experience—people giving advice on how they knew this and that person recovered from a stroke using some natural remedy.

He used to be a fisherman, Don-Don. There was a teacher around my age who they carried every day to shore to bury her body in the sand standing up. It was a community effort. Fishermen volunteered to dig a hole for her before going out to sea. The teacher allegedly did it every day for a month and got well. The teacher still limped, but she got well. My mom was eager to try everything, so I knew I was going down some hole in the sand.

Don-Don and Rivera alternately dug a hole for me in the sand for me to burrow myself in. I gingerly stepped inside the hole and let them cover it with sand until my waist. It felt unnaturally comforting. I didn't feel claustrophobic. I felt very grounded, stable, safe, and supported. I figured that it must be how it feels being inside a womb. Nature spurt me out. I assumed it held the secret of how to heal me.

I didn't bake inside. It was neither hot nor cold. I didn't feel a million sand particles scrape my skin. Sometimes, I would feel the ground shaking, like an earthquake bubbling up from under the earth. The earth throbbed against my legs. I could feel its pulse.

I would stay in the sand twice a day, about an hour each time. Once when the sun was just risen and once as it was going down. How ludicrously grand an experience to be stuck in the ground and to stare at the changing landscape before me. It was like watching a moving painting. Never in my old life would I have found myself literally and figuratively in an experience like that. The wind would caress my face. The waves would make a soothing background noise.

After letting myself out of the hole, I would explore the shore like a kid. For the longest time since I could remember, I would take one look at the sea on vacations and seeing that the tide was low, would decide against swimming. Perhaps I wanted something instantaneous. I wanted the sea large and full, ready for me to swim in like a backyard pool. But that fulness is only a facet of the sea, I learned. It is as full as when it is bare. *What are you made of when you are bare?* The sea seemed to taunt me.

I walked over sand bars, small shallow pools of water, clayish sand, and kelp. There were small white fish and interesting corals if one looked close enough. As I hobbled over the sea floor, I felt like the sea was teaching me more than walking. It was teaching me to listen to the whole call of the sea. It seemed vast and bare yet not empty. Before the stroke, my life was full of minutiae, but I was empty.

Beyond the sandbar, there was this pool of clear shallow water, with powdery sand just before the waters turned dark. It was as if it was just waiting for me. The security guard on duty, Akim, carried a chair for me in the middle of the sea floor. I sat on it, and as if doing the bucket challenge, dipped an empty plastic water bottle and poured sea water on my head. I shrieked in cold delight. It was a picture of simple childlikeness.

One afternoon, as the sun was going down, and I was half buried and the tide was high, I watched Kim try to stand-up paddle. She was trying to balance as the waves roared past her. The image stuck to me, and I clung to it. Here we were, one year to the day when I got the stroke, finally enjoying what the world had to offer. If I didn't get the stroke, I would be hard-pressed to think that we would find ourselves here. Finally, she could enjoy something just for herself, with nothing to think about except for how in a split second the waves might try to outbalance her. I watched my mother, reduced to jitters after the trauma of my experience, take off her shoes, step into the sand and water. I could feel her fists unclenching with her every laugh. We had made it. Finally, we had made it.

72

I returned to the resort a week after I left it. I loved it that much. There was a lure of nature that was compelling. I met the sun a few more times, the skies becoming a watercolour blur of pink and orange by the second. Minutes too late and I would have missed the free display of colours that presented itself to me every morning. *How many have I missed in my lifetime?*

After the sun was settled high up, I would go to the shore and bury myself in the sand with nothing showing but my head, as if a soccer baseball resting on its plate. We had made a peculiar mark at the beach—this bunch of people setting up camp early every morning. A veteran member of its staff, Arnel, who survived a stroke waited for us at the shore one day. He was the first stroke victim I saw who walked without a trace of a stroke in him. The community had thought he was dead, but he resurfaced walking without a limp and with arms fully extended to his side, not crumpling up, closely attached to the trunk as is common in other stroke victims. Out of fear he'd become like one of the stroke victims he always jokingly bullied, he tied a rope from one coconut tree to another, slid his good arm over it, and practiced walking forward. He offered to give me a balm made with *gabon* leaves infused with used oil from a kerosene lamp and coconut vinegar. I was to apply it with a gentle massage to my immobile limbs every night. I applied the oil nightly until I seemed to have used up the oil that only the vinegar remained. I reeked every night before I went to bed. Someone advised to collect seawater, boil it at night, and wipe it across my affected arm and leg. Indigenous advice usually came with an impassioned account of recovery and with unbreakable conviction. We tried everything. If I did not smell like vinegar, I smelled like shellfish. We rubbed these concoctions on my limbs until a better concoction presented itself.

When the sea was full, I would go brave it. A lifeguard would throw a life buoy in the middle of the sea for me to hang on to tightly. I had no means of saving myself if I let go, but somehow the water was kind to my unfolding body. I would drift with the tides until I would find myself at the opposite side of the shore and with the sun high up. The sea eliminated gravity and the fears of land for me; I was flying.

Akim, a kind-hearted guard we had come to know at the resort, suggested that I bury myself horizontally under the sand, so we tried that method as well. A four-year old kid with gorgeous curly hair happened to be at the beach at the same time. He was there to scavenge for baby octopuses, seashells, and other creatures exposed by the low tides. He was a lone ranger amidst a vast playground, serious about his business, with an adventurer's bucket hat as if to emphasize the seriousness of his endeavour. He passed by me as I was halfway buried under the sand. He inquired what we were doing. I answered I was crippled and was burying my limbs in the hopes that the sand will help them move in the future. I expected him to worm uncomfortably on 'crippled', as I was used to receive such reaction from adults, but he didn't flinch. His reaction was refreshing. He wanted to be playfully buried in the sand as well. I was nothing different to him, crippled as I was. His curiosity did not zero in on my sickness, but how it must feel under the sand.

Ezra became a fast friend at the beach. Kim scavenged with him while the tides were low, as I sat in my plastic chair in the middle of the wet, clayish sand. I saw a baby octopus for the first time, jiggly and slimy in his tiny hand. Ezra intuitively knew if you were scared of the octopus. He would thrust it at your face and follow you around in a teasing manner. I held a baby octopus in my hands for the first time. It felt cool. It felt almost friendly. I felt close to and in commune with nature.

Ezra caught a jellyfish, transparent, which he kept in a plastic dipper. Kim recounted that she was previously stung by a jellyfish which led Ezra to excitedly exclaim, 'I was, too!' He seemed incredulous that Kim survived her encounter. 'You're still alive?' he asked with large questioning eyes. Kim solemnly nodded. 'Did you pray too?' Kim solemnly nodded a second time. He was priceless, that kid.

He continued to scavenge as if the sun did not perturb him, as if it was the most natural thing in the world. It actually fed his energy. His dipper slowly filled with creatures of all kinds. Meanwhile, I sat on my chair while my mom poured seawater on top of my head with a broken plastic receptacle. To make things easier for us, Ezra's nanny transferred Ezra's growing collection to a basin and lent us Ezra's dipper. When Ezra saw my mom using the dipper to pour seawater over my head, his eyes widened in horror. He thought all his hard work poured out on top of my head. When we reassured him that his prized collection was safe and sound, he breathed a sigh of relief. The adults had a good laugh over the travails of our young adventurer. He taught us richly of what kids only knew that morning. When we parted ways, he shouted back his address in the city and when he would be back to the beach. Such trust; there was no second-guessing. I wished we could keep that view of the world as we grew older.

When the sun was going down, we set up to horizontally bury myself under the sand a second time during the day. It was a team effort. My family, including my aunts and uncles and cousins, lined themselves up on the shore as I soaked up my surroundings at dusk. I was right in front of the sea. I could hear the roar of the waves. I could smell the foam of the sea. I could feel the cool wind gently blow over my face. A few inches more and the water would have reached my toes. There were two rainbows in the horizon. I didn't even know there could be two rainbows. It was an absurd situation. I never would have found myself in that situation before the stroke. I keep saying it only because it is true. We could enjoy nature before but only on a momentary respite. We never let it take centre stage. What event could bring a moment like this if not for the stroke? I did not feel deprived being hours away from the city where the hospitals were. I did not feel insecure being so far away from Singapore which held all the keys to my rehabilitation. Nature more than compensated for all that the city gave and could have given me. I was being embraced in the most organic way possible.

* * *

My birthday finally arrived. I had spent my previous birthday stuck in my dark hospital room half-conscious. My cousins surprised me with ice cream made in the surrounding sleepy town and stored in old-school tin tubs lined with ice and salt. We shared it with the resort's staff. I liked my party. It was wholesome and with just the right amount of verve for me. We had it in purple yam and cheese flavours. Dr Lee would have been proud.

I went around town for my birthday. The whole place could be scoured under ten minutes. I loved that we were forced to be limited with our choices. There were only two restaurants in town, and one was a pretty long drive away. There was only one fast food joint and one familiar pharmacy and bakery. It made life very simple. I chose to get a haircut on my birthday. I hadn't had one since before the stroke and not one by a professional since the pandemic. We found a nice, tiny salon, only a couple of days old in town. My haircut was under $3, but I loved it. For dinner, I ordered my simple favourites to go from a nearby restaurant. We ordered a modest cake in old-school mocha flavour. I went back to the resort feeling satisfied.

A cart drove me to the resort's restaurant where we set to have my birthday dinner. On the way to the restaurant, drums started beating. Unsuspecting, I rode calmly on the cart. Little did I know that the drums were for me. There was a small band marking my arrival. It was a laughingstock of an entrance. Because it was just after February, all the preparation seemed to be for Valentine's. There was an elaborate dinner set-up at the beach. Apparently, the one the staff was installing at breakfast this morning was for me. One surprise followed another. In the middle of the ceremony and just when I was about to dig into my dinner, rain fell unapologetically. Its timing was perfect. *Yes, wash me clean. Thoroughly, if you must.* I waited as people scrambled to find a way to get me on covered ground, but I didn't mind the rain. The sky never felt so gracious to me. Music blared through the speakers just as I felt the first patter of rain. As much as I was deprived of a birthday last year, I was endowed one this year. My cousins even arranged fireworks *a la* New Year's and a fire dance for the evening. Apparently, they were faced with limited last-minute options in the resort. It reminded me of my previous law firm's Christmas party. There was a celebration of life that was unimaginable. Birthdays never had a special significance for me. It always felt part of a monotonous dance. But I guess when you almost lose your life, a birthday can be very spiritual. I wrote Dr Lee upon my discharge, *I will be always grateful for you every year that I live.* I was a year older. I now know what that entailed.

73

Will didn't come too early for me. Perhaps it exists in the upper echelons of the mind. I couldn't understand what they saw in me—that I had a fighting spirit. I couldn't detect a whiff of it in me. Every time I lay on my hospital bed, I couldn't concern myself with anything except the next episode of the show I was watching on Netflix. I couldn't move my limbs, but I couldn't think of anything else but the trivial.

I wrote to my doctor that I had no fighting spirit except when I had nothing left to give. It was only when my barrel was empty that I was forced to cough up something I didn't know I had within me. Never did I know that I had that capacity—to move something that plainly didn't move. There was a silent acceptance to my immobility, but there was such expectant waiting surrounding me. People were waiting on the impossible that they birthed the possible out of the impossible. *That is how mountains are moved, not instantaneously with the dramatic flick of a finger.* My recovery came with a fealty that translated itself to dedication. I felt like I was in elementary school with a string of classes to attend every day. I longed for a semestral break. My 'classmates' seemed to have escaped rehab one way or another.

About a year after my stroke when my right hand had considerably softened, I took a shower entirely by myself while Kim looked on to see if I needed help. It was taxing on my left arm, which almost had to do everything. I would lean down from my shower chair to scrub my legs and feet while making sure

I didn't slide out of my seat. The process took very long and spent all my mental energies. I could feel my mind sweat as it tried to ingrain new patterns in it. I had grown accustomed to being bathed and to see bath time as a relaxing slice of time. But that first time I held the shower head back showed me what I could do. It, or whatever it was that needed to be done, did not have to be done for me. I had almost forgotten that I had done things on my own before. I began to scrub parts of my body that were always overlooked. Back in the hospital, I talked myself out of telling the nurse in charge that she missed a spot while bathing me. I convinced myself that the water in the end would wash me clean. If there was soap left on my body, I consoled myself that a towel would wipe it dry anyway. The first time I took a shower, I regained those little liberties that I had given up. *I owned my body after all.* It felt as exhilarating and liberating as spring. I haphazardly dressed myself. It was awkward at first, but it became easier and smoother.

After I had seen what I could do by myself, I thought to walk a few rounds around the house every forty-five minutes. I would turn on the speakers and blare upbeat old school music through them. I would choose a song and aim to finish a round by the time it ended. Then I would pick a shorter song and try to beat my own record. *Two minutes and forty-five seconds. Two minutes and fifteen seconds.* We loved dancing to Beyoncé's 'The Best Thing I Never Had' and Marvin Gaye and Tammi Terrell's 'Ain't No Mountain High Enough'. My mom and sister were complicit in the whole thing. We danced as if on a Choo Choo train, with me awkwardly dancing like a stick figure.

Then I would try the ballads. They calmed me unexpectedly, making me fall into step with the rhythm of the song. My jerky movements slowly smoothed themselves out with the soft strums of the song.[9] I caught myself taking rhythmic steps for the first

---

[9] Please don't expect normal walking.

time while the melancholic hums of 'Have I Told You Lately' played. It was a happy moment of reckoning. I kept silent so as not to ruin the moment. It was 30 April, just a little over a year after I got the stroke. I couldn't have been more elated. It turns out that when you walk long enough, you give your brain enough time to consolidate all the information it picks up along the way until it can pull itself together. I just always conveniently hobbled to where I needed to go before. Apparently, it was not enough. I silently played the tune of 'Have I Told You Lately' in my head as a metronome to make me to walk.

Learning to walk was much like spinning a top and not making it stop. I had to balance my trunk on my legs, and they were constantly moving. In my body, there seemed to be this heavy bowling ball that veered easily to the left or the right and which I had to keep at centre so I would not fall. However, I had to shift the weight from one leg to another every time I needed to take a step so I could lift the forward-moving leg. In other words, every step involved a split-second one-legged stand. The technicalities were mind-boggling, plus I didn't have enough body awareness to keenly know where my body parts were. Dragging my affected leg felt like dragging an inanimate part of my body until my knees softened, and I felt safe bearing weight on it.

Siva always had the mantra, *think faster, execute slower*. I wondered how to do that. But as I kept on walking, I found that my brain could summarize a series of commands into one unified command. Usually that command was to do something functional. All my segmented instructions on how to walk, I found, could be incorporated in a single *Forward!* All my body parts seemed to work together as if on cue upon that command. I also found that once I've mastered all the segmented parts, I should just leave my body and brain to do its magic together. There's a right combination of body and brain that works. The brain has to take a step back and let the body lead where it thinks is best.

About one year and two months after my discharge, I took off my foot splint which I wore while walking. I needed the splint to keep my toes level to the ground. Otherwise, my foot just dropped. I thought about all those ballet dancers who had to balance on their toes. I essentially had to be able to do that to walk without a splint. That was a near impossible challenge, so we concentrated instead on raising my ankle higher and higher. In the early days, it took three people to push my ankle to form a ninety-degree angle. Wherever did my ankle get the strength that it had? I, for sure, could not fight three people. It was like playing and winning tug-of-war without me even trying.

After a lot of stretches and wearing the night splint judiciously every night, my foot flattened to a degree that I could drag it on the floor without a splint. My ankle would twist to its sides, forever scaring us of a sprain, but it was the only way to go. Coach would always warn us, 'use extreme caution.' I didn't know the right balance between stretching myself and keeping myself safe. I would walk with a gait belt tied around my waist held by a person at my back, like a dog on a leash. Simultaneously, I would wear a band around my waist which someone pulled to simulate an incline while wearing a 1-kilo weight on my bad ankle. Later, we felt confident enough to get the gait belt off.

With the splint off, slowly, I felt that the ground beneath my feet was something familiar, not plastic. It brought me back to the land I trod on before the stroke and all that it carried. Walking became more familiar. I didn't have to think too hard. It was like my feet remembered. I walked barefoot on grass and stubbed my toes on the earth. When I stubbed them successively, the earth told my toes to lift them up as I stepped to avoid the pain of stubbing them. As a reflex, my toes straightened themselves out when it could take the pain no longer to make way for the ground. It was wonderful seeing the reflex. The earth and the body just seemed to talk directly between themselves. I remembered seeing hordes of people walking barefoot in the Singapore airport. It was my first time to see people barefoot in such a metropolis. I had grown up seeing people in shoes, but maybe that was the original design. Wouldn't our feet teach us best how to walk? It was the best idea to remove my splint.

I kept a gratitude journal and a drawing book. On the left side of my journal, I would scribble three things I was grateful for with my left hand. Then on the right-hand side, I would draw things with my right. I began with what literally looked like chicken scratch. It was all I could manage with my right. To draw strokes, I thrusted my trunk forward and backward because my arm was tightly attached to my trunk. Somehow, I persevered in what was an extremely frustrating exercise. Little by little, I drew tiny images. My wrist could rotate only a small bit. Every day, I drew as my hand allowed me until I enjoyed my newfound creativity. I looked forward to what I would draw the next day.

I ran my bookstore in the small pockets of time I had in between therapy sessions. I once read that Teddy Roosevelt interested himself in so many extracurricular activities that he had to do schoolwork in between activities with 'blistering intensity'.[10] I always wondered what that meant. I tried to apply it to the way I worked before the stroke, but I didn't really know what it meant until after. I found that I could do so much more with my hour than I ever did before. Maybe 'blistering intensity' was borne out of necessity. On most days, I only had an hour to ninety minutes to myself. In the law firm, we used to slave away until the wee hours of the day to finish a memorandum. We would finish (and consequently, have peace of mind) after but at the extreme cost of time and energy. We would be like floating zombies by morning. This time, I had my full brain on my side, and what a feeling it was! We always know how to live optimally but somehow always succumb to poorer choices.

---

[10] Newport, C. (2016). *Deep Work* (1st ed.). Grand Central Publishing.

My uncle sent a reflexologist from his hometown to do acupressure on me daily for a month. I got even busier. I now had occupational therapy, physiotherapy, walking, and acupressure amidst all other minor exercises. I got two hours of acupressure every day. The second day, I felt like jelly and did not know where to get the energy for my other very physical therapies. My limbs were doused with very hot water twice a day, and I took steam baths every other day.

I was wary of placebo. I had learned a thing or two during my acupuncture phase. I was careful not to attribute certain progress to a certain form of therapy no matter the accompanying testimony because the truth was, I was a hodgepodge of therapies. I didn't know what worked because I did everything concurrently. We were willing to try anything that claimed to accelerate my progress.

I read my daily Bible passages out loud. I sang my Do-Re-Mis and even rap songs. I blew on the spirometer multiple times daily. My caregiver pulled on my face, as if intent on creating premature wrinkles on my face.

I swam during the weekends. Dr Lee once told me that I would enjoy the water. In it, I could try new movements without people staring at me. I could try to balance without fear of falling. The water would envelope me. The first few times in the water, I could barely put my feet flat on the pool floor that I had to wear my splint and sandal underwater with weights tied around my bad ankle.

I found that I could no longer hold my breath underwater. My mouth, nostrils, and lungs didn't seem to know yet how to co-ordinate themselves. The first time I tried dunking myself under water, I coughed hysterically. It was odd that something I fully knew how to do, I could not do any more. I bought floaters to carry my trunk while I attempted to paddle and kick away. My family helped me to lay on my back and just stare at the blue of the skies.

One night, way past midnight, I woke feeling the urge to pee. I called on my caregiver. I whispered and then bellowed her name about twenty times but to no avail. Kim was fast asleep too. With no other choice, I pulled my commode closer to my bed. I stood on wobbly legs, relying mostly on my left. My right ankle couldn't yet rest flat on the floor. Without a splint, I carefully pivoted and positioned myself in front of the commode, pulled down my pyjamas (balancing the hell out of me), aware that if I were to fall, break something, and risk more than a year of therapy, no one would save me. When I managed to successfully slide down the commode and do my business, I realized that I could not get back up, pull up my pyjamas, turn to remove the attached bucket and dump it into the washroom, which was many steps and obstacles away. But even so, as I sat there in that quiet, dark moment with the whole world sleeping, I realized that it was the first time I was truly alone. *This is how independence looks like. This is how I regain it.* I went back to bed exhilarated.

Learned wilfulness (I'm not really sure if there is a term like that) is a beautiful thing. It is a powerful antidote to learned helplessness. I learned to set goals because I saw that the ends that I yearned for were reachable. I was then the hare; now I am the slow and steady tortoise, and it is okay. It made me want to do things myself, not at the urging of others. Getting a stroke is like being lost in the dark. Neuroplasticity is having someone, finally after what feels like eons, turn on a lightbulb.

I don't know what to feel about the Silver Spring monkeys from my own country that were brutally experimented on to discover that our brain could develop new pathways to relearn a certain movement. I saw a photo of a monkey, being tied on all fours while parts of its brain were deactivated, to see if it could wake up the thought-of dead parts of its brain. I saw a picture of the monkey with its good arm on a sling to prevent it from using it. The monkey could very well be me. That is how they do therapy even today. They sling the good arm so that the stroke victim would be forced to use his or her bad arm and develop new neural pathways in the process. The experiments were cruel, and they also saved my life.

Will doesn't show itself until you are willing to do more than you think you could do. I remember being on sand dunes at one of the ruined ancient gates of the Silk Road. The wind was lashing. It was biting cold, with the air sharply breezing through the bare windows of the old jade gates. I looked at the way back we had to traverse to get back to our bus. It was a painfully long, bare stretch of desert land. Will came to me in a similar moment. I had finally gone out of my house's gate to the streets to build my endurance. I reached the first lamppost which we used as an indicator of how far I had gone the day before. I looked back to the way home. It was half a kilometre downhill on rugged concrete. I was so spent. I could almost laugh or cry if I expended more energy, but I had to go home just as I had to walk. Some things required no explanation like that. A part of you just needs you, and you submit with no excuses.

74

This account would not be written without my family by my side. Literally, they were with me every step of the way. I remember we used to walk in the garden of our apartment in Singapore at snail's pace at the curiosity of the other apartment dwellers. We would trudge all the way through the hallway to the elevator to our apartment door, with them forming a human wall around me, taking for as long a time as we needed.

They put their lives on hold. Theirs is a case of selfless devotion I got to learn firsthand. My mother acted as if her life's work vanished, and she had to rebuild again. Kim willingly carried my yoke. I can only imagine it to be extremely heavy, but she did it in a way that I never felt indebted to her. I was her only cause for being even long into my recovery. My dad refused to go home to the Philippines so he could accompany me to therapy when it was the most boring chore to do. Mimi cut short her time abroad under scholarship to help me through my confinement. I wouldn't have then thought it fair pre-stroke, but love knows and admits no other way.

When I say they are relentless, they *are* relentless, to the point of my discomfort. My mom has an iron will, and it's not always pleasant, especially if it doesn't match my own sometimes. If she could live vicariously through me just so she could exercise all hours of the day, she would. But because perhaps of my family's drive beyond normal, I can look forward to a good recovery.

They made sure I could get the best life back in all circumstances. The whole experience changed us.

I wrote Dr Lee in my first follow-up visit with him after returning to Singapore:

Dear Dr Lee,

I couldn't very well come here without a letter. It would be like entering a train without a ticket.

I could have ended my story upon discharge or upon returning home. I would have been satisfied (It appears that when you've gotten a stroke, you can do no wrong). But I'm glad I didn't, or I wouldn't have completely learned what I needed to learn through this ordeal. Love of family can be painfully human but fiercely enduring.

I said in so many words what you taught me before. It seemed so absurd that you only went out one weekend while you were in Boston because your wife was left behind here with the kids. But in fact, that's what my family did for me. Somewhere along my journey, I wanted them desperately to have a life, for me not to be the centre of the universe, but I guess in some universes, love does not permit that. I have a lot to learn now, but I have to hold out because as you said, he who laughs last, laughs best.

May we all have a good laugh after this season. You witnessed my time to sow; you shall share in my time to reap. So, what's next?

Kind regards,

Tracy

75

I know I am extremely privileged to spend eight months of my convalescence in Singapore. The place nursed me back to health. I thought how casual it was for Singaporeans not to feel insecure about health care. A person can get a stroke and feel ensured that he or she would be brought to a stroke-ready hospital, or his or her finances be taken care of. We didn't have that privilege back home.

Mae, my aide, who had resumed to take care of me from my caregiver spoke of a neighbour she had back home. That neighbour was allegedly berated by doctors and therapists because he impregnated his wife who had just suffered a stroke. How was a woman unable even to control her bladder, order her uterus, soon after the stroke, to excrete a child? The wife allegedly couldn't speak. Could she have given consent? Was she actually in a sound mind to give consent? She would have been like a statue. How hopeless a situation must one be in to not care about the consequences of an act? I found myself looking at the legal and humane side of the situation.

If I weren't brought to Singapore, would I have a second life? What kind of life could I look forward to? I was brought to the best hospital in our city. It was even famous throughout the country. If it wasn't stroke-ready, which hospital was? If it supposedly was stroke-ready, its stroke-readiness could not save a life or at least the essence of it. I began thinking of ways to change things. In what alternate universe—if I were home—could I have achieved an outcome that Singapore gave me? For sure, at one point in my life, I wanted to pack up and leave, live in a place that could save me. But there was so much to be done here. While the grass was certainly greener in many ways outside, it seemed just plainly greener to me, but I was unexplainably content in my brown burnt soil.

Mae had to leave for work abroad after a few months. I had gotten close to her. I wanted upward mobility for her, and I understood her leaving was the most direct way towards it. I couldn't deprive her of that opportunity. She was going to Saudi. She had a five-year old. I asked if he was okay with her leaving. She said that he was hesitant at first, but that he finally agreed to her leaving in exchange for a life-size toy car—the big ones you could find at the department store. A childhood with a mother and a toy car. He seemed to have gotten the short end of the stick. I should think he wasn't fully aware of all the details of his bargain. If I were the mother, I didn't know whether to be happy or sad that my kid finally agreed to my stint away. What has my country come to? It pained me that many in my homeland had to make these choices.

We ate one last time at our usual Friday night haunt. She barely touched her falafels. Funny that it should be a staple to where she was heading. We dug in the millet and smoothies made from cocoas and cayenne peppers, food and drink I would not have touched pre-stroke, but here I was frequenting the place almost every week. The world was moving endlessly before me, as I was working on myself. She was passing. I marked a period of her transitory life, like a pin on a giant map. We said our hearty goodbyes. I gave her a book, *Paddington*, for her five-year old and a bracelet for her leaving. She asked me what I wanted from Saudi. I meant to give my gifts stoically but broke into a sob upon saying my goodbyes. I still could not hold my emotion. While my mind and my heart understood fully that she had to leave, something primitive in me just had to break loose. It was difficult to be taken seriously with my loud, uncontrolled outbursts. My grown-up side could not be taken apart from its noisy, childish half. I was embarrassed to say the least, but I felt attached to her in a way I did not expect.[11]

---

[11] Mae eventually chose to stay in the Philippines.

76

It was time. I was ready to look at the mass of messages that accumulated since I was in the ICU. I remember a guy in rehab who had gone back to work a few days a week. He had remarked about the ton of unread email that awaited him at his return. Numbering thousands, it nearly overwhelmed him. I didn't hope to back-read all my emails. I was quite happy having skipped all of them. I remember being particularly bogged down by messages in various messaging apps before the stroke. At one unthinking push of a forward button, a person unnecessarily took up space in my brain. Even if I barely opened trivial messages, the collective number of them weighed heavily on me.

I had to open my messages in Messenger though. There were people who worried about me. I opened the app. *There was my life before.* It felt ethereal. There was a barrage of interrupted conversations. I scrolled back to the day I was admitted. The messages plunged me back to the dark days of the ICU. *Who was the first person who knew I was admitted? Who cared beyond the ordinary?* I read as Kim updated my friends, obviously clinging to whatever silver lining there was. I keenly regarded the time stamps of the conversations. It objectively retraced the events that unfolded. There was a thorough update to friends that I had two strokes, that I was recovering, but then they found out I had another stroke. That piece of information didn't immediately settle with me. It jolted me out of the story that I had clearly laid out for myself after the stroke.

I confronted Kim about what I'd just read. They *had* known about the third stroke in the Philippines but had opted not to tell me. I had another stroke, after all, when I told them I could interlace my fingers no longer. I was right. I wasn't hallucinating. In fact, I had four strokes. I let that piece of information sink in me slowly. 'Approximately one third of those who suffer a stroke will die, often from a second or third subsequent assault on the neurological system.'[12] The Philippine hospital was not sorely incompetent; I was just severely unlucky.

My closest friends obviously received the news in shock. It was odd reading some of the messages. Some seemed to mourn me already. They recounted what kind of person I was and the relationship we shared. I was still alive, but they were realistic about the situation. When was I getting out of the ICU anyway not resembling a vegetable? How long were they supposed to hold on to the version of me they knew when obviously that person no longer existed? It would have been unfair to make them care for me for as long as I was breathing through a tube.

---

[12] McCrum, R. (1999). *My Year Off.* Broadway Books.

77

I suppose I have to give a rumination about death here having come so close to it. Robert McCrum in *My Year Off,* an autobiographical account of his experience with stroke, described his brush with death thus: 'I have not lost my respect, of course, but I have lost my fear. I know what it feels like to be carried away, helpless, towards oblivion and finding by great fortune the current slow and swirl towards the bank, leaving me sprawled, quite helpless, on a new shore.'

To be honest, I did not think of death, other than probably on my second day in the ICU in the Philippines when I was losing my vision and my voice. I had motioned a wave goodbye with my right hand to my family when it was fast weakening. I was clearly degenerating. I didn't know what else I was bound to lose in the near future and to what extent I could still lose it before turning off the lights. In extremis, I found myself practical rather than sentimental. My mom didn't understand what I was trying to say, but Kim did, and she stubbornly refused it. Plainly rejected it. After that, I harboured no more thoughts of death. I was drawn to the bouts of procedures I was subjected to. I didn't any more actively participate in my own life as much as I was subject to it.

Despite the difficulties and the intense hardship of being stuck immobile (my body was my own prison), I did not wish me dead. I was effectively a limp vegetable, but even then I did not think my life was meaningless. I was angry with God, for sure. C.S. Lewis once wrote about this feeling of forsakenness in *A Grief Observed* as quoted in *My Year Off*: 'Meanwhile, where is God? This is one of the most disquieting symptoms. When you are happy, so happy that you have no sense of needing Him, so happy that you are tempted to feel His claims upon you as an interruption, if you remember your self and turn to Him with gratitude and praise, you will be—or so it feels—welcomed with open arms. But go to Him when your need is desperate, when all other help is in vain, and what do you find? A door slammed in your face, and a sound of bolting, and double bolting on the inside. After that, silence.' Maybe that is the cross. Maybe I had to experience the low point before being actually lifted up. Maybe my feet had to touch the ground for me to know how it is to be off it. Faith is not made of the easy stuff, but I learned that He is faithful when He says, 'When you pass through the waters, I will be with you.' (Isaiah 43:2) He sat by my hospital bed when I had to carry my cross. I realized that even He was not exempt from the feeling of human forsakenness when He endured His own cross.

Two things were abundantly clear while I was strapped to my hospital bed. The future seemed bright. By the measure of my suffering, I knew my reward was going to be great. Second, there was inexplicable joy in my suffering. I did not feel alone; rather, I felt embraced, like I had a steady companion who made everything better. I knew with a strange confidence that for those willing to see it, He endows a silver lining to the most extremes of suffering. There was joy in the sorrow, rejoicing in the weeping, no matter how ironic it felt. Maybe the feeling was borne out of knowing I had survived a fatal blow. That should have made me appreciate life more, but I didn't have that feeling overwhelmingly. What I felt overwhelmingly was steady companionship.

For sure, I had my low points. There were the angry bouts just because of how difficult the easy things were. There was the self-pity state, my being resigned to my fate after seeing how my deficits consumed me. But thank God, I didn't have them often enough to consume me whole. Maybe I didn't have to have the will early on. I just needed not to give up.

78

I wrote the first ever entry in our reading club at Blithe Books, *The Tortoise and the Hare*, published on Instagram on 29 May 2023:

The Tortoise and The Hare

Entry No. 1:

My Year Off by Robert McCrum

Robert McCrum was forty-two when he suffered a debilitating stroke which left his left side totally paralysed, his speech impaired, and his sense of self radically altered. He was then editor-in-chief at Faber and Faber.

I liked how he described his brush with death: 'I have not lost my respect, of course, but I have lost my fear. I know what it feels like to be carried away, helpless, towards oblivion and finding by great fortune the current slow and swirl towards the bank, leaving me sprawled, quite helpless, on a new shore.' It reminds me of John Donne's 'Death, Be Not Proud'. Or that 1 Corinthians passage, 'O death, where is thy sting? O grave, where is thy victory?'

We usually think of a heart attack as fatal but stroke, as not so. He says: 'Everyone, for instance, knows about heart attacks, but a "brain attack" or stroke, can wreak just as much havoc, and in many different dimensions. The heart stops in only one way, but the brain has several ways to remind us of human frailty.' Indeed, a fully functioning brain underpins the flourishing of the mind, and the mind is me.

I can't believe that at the time he had a stroke, neuroplasticity was yet undiscovered. I don't know how my hope could have fanned out if all the experts knew then was that the mind was immutable. Immutable essentially meant immobile, among other deficits. Who would have known that my country would have made a consequential contribution to my recovery through the Silver Spring monkeys, despite the controversy surrounding them? It is hard to believe that physiotherapy was seen as akin to water divining and herbal therapy when it is seen as the cornerstone of recovery now.

A lot of time has passed from when he had his stroke up to now, but the insight to human experience remains as universal, stark, and true. Perhaps through the commonality of experience, I sped through this one. A hare kind of read.

Note: the book is personal; not currently in our collection

#thetortoiseandtheharereadingclub

79

I met Lola when her family invited me to a private painting class they had organized for her after surviving an open-heart surgery. She was frail and thin in her wheelchair, but she did not seem at the edge of despair. Prior to her surgery, she felt nothing unusual. In fact, she was set to go off to college. During a routine admissions check-up, the doctors found that she had an enlarged aorta. Her syndrome had apparently found a way to catch up with her. She had Marfan syndrome, an illness that causes uneven growth in the limbs, looseness of the joints, and a tendency to develop aneurysms, especially in the aorta.

When the doctors found out about her enlarged aorta, they said there was no time to waste. They had to open her up in the fastest time possible. After the surgery, she felt unexplainable pain in her legs. She walked gingerly with a walker. Her legs had nothing to do with her illness and surgery, yet here they were robbing her of her life. They put her on morphine because of the pain. Prior to the surgery, while possibly closer to death, she felt like a normal person.

While not at the edge of despair, she was inching towards it. I could feel it. I met her two weeks after her surgery. I did not want the rest of her life to drain away from her. I wanted her to hold fast to it. She had to know she had control over losing it. She could own her mind before it could mercilessly own her. She was much too young to succumb to fate. She was almost half my age. I thought myself young in this business, but here she was. I felt ages older and felt a responsibility to relay what had helped me to a fellow soldier.

Learning she loved fantasies and adventure, I gave her *Dune* by Frank Herbert, *The Left Hand of Darkness* and *The Wizard of Earthsea* by Ursula Le Guin. If only I had a book for every known form of suffering. I wanted the books to keep her afloat.

I did not see Lola until two weeks after our last painting session in her house. I invited her to my home to paint. I wanted to thank her for adding a dimension to my life that I would not have had had she not opened her home to me, then virtually a stranger. (It is difficult to receive the world when you are still in the process of receiving yourself). I was surprised to see that she had requested to get some takeout enroute my home. She had specifically asked for spring rolls. She was in considerably high spirits and painted beautifully.

I could not pretend I knew her business. She was in an entirely different ball game. But I saw myself in her in what she had to hurdle. Suffering, bearing a different face, is still suffering.

80

I learned about forbearance, ironically, in oil painting class. It is easy to say one has forgiven, but is not as easy to say one has forbore. To hold back when one feels in the right (rightly or wrongly), you'd think that'd be an easy job for someone who has been rewarded a second life out of nowhere, but it is not so easy after all. Not if you're on the losing end. I guess magnanimity is not intuitive for everyone.

I painted with my left. When the instructor learned that I had to paint with my non-dominant left hand, he remarked, 'We're going to be doing abstract art with you.' My left managed with surprising dexterity. I never relied on it for anything significant before. I thus never knew the potential of this equal half of my body that I had lugged around all my life. I was shocked at the result. My left produced a painting my right could never have produced, even when fully able as it was before. It was like I unlocked a side of my brain never revealed to me before. *Did I become more creative after the stroke?* It was the first time I wasn't relearning something from scratch. I would have learnt as a beginner even if I didn't get a stroke. I found myself in the only time I was apace with my old self. I could feel my brain breathe, exhale.

'Don't be afraid to go outside the lines,' the instructor chimed. 'You can always cover it up with another coat of paint.' I liked that oil painting was so forgiving, so fluid, and not linear. The more mistakes you made, the prettier your painting seemed to get; the more colours you mixed, the more real and vivid your painting became. I liked that no matter how people could mess up your painting, you knew you always had the power to make it your own in the end. You couldn't always revert it to the original, but you could do something fresh about it.

It is hard to forbear when you think of your life as radically and permanently affected by outside elements. It is hard to forbear when people unwittingly consume too much of something as exhaustible as your life.[13] People unknowingly or knowingly make dents in your one life. But I am not a watercolour painting, I learned that afternoon. I was made of oil.

---

[13] To what extent do we own our lives, if at all, and to what extent are we mere stewards in this long continuum we are part of? Or perhaps there is no such dilemma? The two choices are actually one?

81

My occupational therapist, who was always reliable and an Energizer Bunny, suddenly had bouts of absence. It was unlike her. She had migraines. She felt tired after every session of ours, but she chalked it up to her hectic lifestyle. One day, the doctor recommended that she have an MRI scan. When a couple of days after her scan, she failed to come, I knew something was wrong.

On our next session, she showed me her scan. Unlike mine, the scan was immediately understandable to the layman. There was a huge white cyst taking up the space for her spinal cord, such that the thin cord so vital to life was squeezed in its narrow chamber under extreme pressure. It caused numbness in her face and left arm, which made me to prompt, 'Those were my symptoms!' But nothing fazed Pria. She was as unperturbed as a zen master. Even then, she still resumed sessions while waiting for her surgery and drove herself long distances out of town.

Immediately, after knowing her results, I felt myself turn solicitous, concerned. *How odd that I should have this feeling again after the stroke.* I had been so used to being the sick one. I so craved to be treated normally, but here I was being exactly what I hated for Pria. *How odd that this woman who had steadily brought me back to life was at the verge of possibly suffering a fate like mine?* Symptoms for illnesses in the spine mirrored closely that of injuries to the brain.

Her impending surgery hit too close to home.

82

With Pria gone for a few weeks, I enlisted my young deaf cousin to playfully hold the fort. He seemed extra caring, compared to other kids. He wore a kindness about him that spoke that he knew disability for a very long time.

What I expected to be child's play turned out to be this very gruelling occupational therapy session. He has never had a session his whole life, but he was keen to pick up my deficits and knew instinctively what to do to make me functional. He adopted a boxing stance and hopped to his feet, exhibiting brisk fisted actions. To adopt his pretence, I swerved, ducked my head, extended my arm to pretend punch, and lifted my legs as if to dance on my feet. It was a perturbation exercise like no other. In fact, it was the most advanced I've had. He taught me how to move my feet methodically. It was weight shifting *à la* Manny Pacquiao.

He then moved to work on my fine motor movements. 'Let me think,' he said solemnly, while imagining what I could do with tiny instruments. He took some exercise putty, of the consistency of clay and slime mixed together, stuck it to one end of a dumbbell, made the dumbbell stand on the table on its sticky side, took a curling rod, and made me bang it on the dumbbell like hitting a brass gong with a stick.

Seeing that the dumbbell stuck sturdily to the table through the putty, he placed putties on both sides of the dumbbell to glue them to the table. Then, he slipped an exercise band along the spine of the dumbbell. I was then to pull hard on the exercise band, extending my stiff arm and activating my core muscles. I've had all my therapists act as the dumbbell for me. He was the only one clever enough to spare himself the effort.

He created a relay for me made from exercise bands, stuck to a table with putty, and shaped like rings. I was to shoot plastic tacks in the rings. The rings were arranged from nearest to farthest from me. To shoot at the farthest rings, I had to extend my heavy right arm straight. I was under time pressure. He placed a toy hourglass before me to ensure that I could dispose of the tacks quickly enough. At the end of the exercise, he mixed up the red and yellow putties, which were for different tactile strength, into an orange one. We had putty stuck stubbornly all over the exercise bands when we finished. I think he mistook the exercise putty with Play-Doh.

He also made a punching bag of himself. I was to box his hands. The routine seemed simple enough until it wasn't. Like in a video game, his hands started moving elevator-like, and I had to catch up to them in order to hit them.

He took his job seriously. He promised his dad that he would go to sleep right after he bought a hand strengthening kit that he found for me online. He knew how to pull his dad to his corner. True to his word, after his dad added the tools to his cart and checked them out, he took off his hearing aid and went straight to bed. We called him Dr Lance. I seriously wanted to end my therapy sessions with my professional therapists in order to move exclusively to him.

83

Kim and I found ourselves alone one quiet evening and decided to watch a movie to relax for the night. We had not had a slow night for so long. While scrolling through television shows and movies, I saw a red ad at the bottom of *Lincoln Lawyer*: 'New episodes'. It was the series we intently watched in the early days in the Singapore hospital. I couldn't believe I had survived to watch another season. I marvelled at the continuity of life.

84

Marco replaced Pria. He said I should come out of every session as if I had just finished a HIIT workout. We worked out for an hour straight with minimal rest. He was not one for small talk. I was not used to that. He reminded me of the first physical therapist I had in the Singapore hospital. We performed manoeuvres that circled me back to that early time in the hospital. *Aah, this was what she wanted to achieve.* I could barely bend my legs then, but she wanted me to kneel on one knee. This time, I could do a one-legged bridge comfortably, but back then the feat had felt impossible.

I realized my physiotherapist then was only bringing out what she could at the earliest possible time. It was just frustrating for me to be told to move a leg, with everyone expectant, when I knew it was plainly not going to move. Perhaps, just trying to think of the process then to create new neural pathways was enough, but I did not know that then. I was used to a limb moving when I asked it to move. I'm sure she had my best interests in mind. I'm sorry that she met me while I was in my rapids. Taking stock of the changes in my body took almost the whole of me.

85

I finally got it. It was like entering a rite of passage. I was terrified. I didn't know how my body would react. If my limbs had to undergo so much therapy every day to remember or relearn how they functioned before, how can my internal body parts do the same, when they have not had a chance to practise? How can I induce them to take their places and fight the virus with me? My mind was willing, but I didn't know if my body was my comrade.

I woke up from a nap as if I had just ingested water through my nose. That's what I made out of it. I didn't remember how a cold felt. Therapy after therapy, the feeling lingered there, until it dawned on me when the feeling seemed to infiltrate my throat like an army of ants. I was going down with a cold.

Reality was much kinder to me than I had anticipated. My reflexes took over. I wondered which hidden part of the brain they come from. I thanked God it was spared from my stroke. I wished my reflex system could cover a much broader area than it did. That it took over everything when I had the stroke and made everything easier.

86

22 August 2023. That was the date when I turned the TV on to watch the news. When I was rushed to the ICU, the Ukraine–Russia war just broke. There was some Oscars hullabaloo on the hospital TV. During therapy in Singapore, my therapists discussed the ugly court battle between Johnny Depp and Amber Heard. I was shocked. I didn't even know they had separated and were hurling crazy accusations against each other. I had lived an artificial life, devoid of anything that hurt, that might bog my broken brain down. But that night, I was ready.

I had heard about the Maui wildfires that consumed the island. I typed 'Maui wildfire' on YouTube. A barrage of videos displayed on my screen. The videos showed apocalyptic scenes I'd only ever seen dramatized in movies. The fires blazed and were coming after people. I thought about my trauma and that despite how severe it had been, another very different form could quite present itself to other people. It was like there was an endless permutation of suffering that could inflict us at any time. I imagined myself to be a character in that apocalyptic scene and didn't know how I could have survived, even as my able self. Suffering in the face. That's what I would call what happened to them.

The Ukraine–Russia war was still on. Almost three years now, it's been on. I thought it was unlikely that world leaders intimately knew suffering. It is doubtful whether they did to inflict so much tragedy. Whatever they are fighting for, is it worth more than life?

I thought how lucky I was that I could afford the time in between before I faced reality. Not everyone is so lucky. Perhaps theirs is a motivation to recover I will never know.

87

The whole time I was recovering, Blithe Books was bleeding. Sales trickled in, and that was being generous. Books were ageing on us as time went on. Yellow dots and streaks scarred the pages of my once beautiful books, as if reminding me of their overtime at my shelf. I was inundated with books I didn't know what to do with. I wanted to keep Blithe Books going. It has helped in more ways than I ever imagined, but I was hesitant to pour in more of my savings in a business running out of gas.

Opening a tiny bookstore is dreamy. It is every bit as whimsical as depicted in the movies. But it is also spelled with beautiful struggle. It was nice in an ironic way to have a problem outside of fixing myself. I was slowly returning to ordinary life, lending my brain to ordinary affairs, unbeknownst to myself. I decided to fill up space in a farmer's market within the city. We brought a small collection of books and displayed them amongst people intent to get their produce for the coming week. They were there for the fresh greens and the eggs, but rent was free. That was good enough for us.

Sales were dismal the first few weeks. I was at a crossroads. *Do I pack up for good or willingly swim through deeper waters?* Seeing that it was impractical for us to wait to garner enough sales at the farmer's market to procure new books, I decided to dive head-long into uncertainty. I placed an order for new books with different suppliers, deciding to breathe fresh life into Blithe. *Why not give it the fight of its life?* I was unsure of many things in my life, but with this one, I never had a doubt.

88

I faced my tablet. Any ordinary concern would have caused me to open it and search for the curious concern on Google. It floundered me that I had never thought to research about what happened to me. The general prognosis of someone who suffered a severe brainstem stroke like mine was dismal, but I seemed sufficiently far from those expectations now. I had beat the odds. I felt sufficiently removed from the assault. I felt ready to inquire about what happened to me.

I first read about another experience similar to mine in *My Year Off*. It was weird reading what happened to me off a page. I now had the luxury of reading about them. Then, I had to live through them. Stroke was the most common cause of death in the Western world, it said. Stroke never held a lethal connotation for me like a heart attack or an aneurysm, but what a killer it apparently was. It said, '(o)f those who survive the initial "insult", about half will be left with permanent severe disability. The physical consequence of stroke is a horrifying catalogue of damage that includes personality changes, impaired sensation, paralysis, incontinence, visual or language problems, deafness, blindness, seizures, and even swallowing difficulties, the distressing manifestations of what the textbooks describe as "neurological deficits".' It is silencing hearing about the deficits, but I had lived vividly through most of them. I breathed a sigh of relief that I didn't suffer from personality change nor deafness.

I had closely escaped locked-in syndrome, where one is immobile everywhere except the eyes. In my early days in the ICU, up to when I was air-lifted to Singapore, I was effectively paralysed on both sides. I had troubled vision. I drooled everywhere. I could not swallow even my own saliva. I shuddered to think what could have happened to me if my left didn't slowly wake up like it did. I was thirty-five; I could have lived the rest of my life like a thinking statue. It felt worse than dying. It amazed me that a French journalist, Jean-Dominique Bauby, with locked-in syndrome still managed to write a book, *The Diving Bell and the Butterfly*, about his predicament. What he wrote was eventually published four days before his death. He memorized in his head what he wanted to say then listened to an assistant read the alphabet for him to spell out each word. He blinked his left eye once at the appropriate letter for yes, twice for no.[14] His achievement was exhilarating, triumphant. It made me see that the brain is this magnificent thing, that the will knows no bounds, that being normal is being spoiled like crazy. I made a mental note to buy the book.

I remember watching *Breathe* in the ICU. The doctors in the film were proud of the stunning technological marvel deep in the German alps that they had invented. It allowed sick people to live longer. The marvel was a room, blinding white, almost antiseptic, with wall-mounted chambers housing quadriplegic patients coffin-like with nothing protruding but their heads. To probably add some sort of stimulation, a mirror was placed opposite the patient's heads so they could see their eyes. The room was filled almost to the ceiling with quadriplegic patients, as if on bunk beds but in an eternal freezer. It was prison upon prison being heaped atop of each other. *What did I do to escape such a fate?*

For the first time, I opened my files from the Philippine hospital. Any piece of information previously withheld from me

---

[14] McCrum, R. (1999). *My Year Off*. Broadway Books.

now lay open. For the first time, I read about words like diplopia, dysarthria, paraesthesia, etc.

> Diplopia—double vision or seeing double. Dysarthria—a motor speech disorder in which the muscles you use to produce speech are damaged, paralysed, or weakened. Paresthesia—a tingling, numbing, or prickling sensation that is usually felt in the arms, legs, or feet, but can also occur in other parts of the body. Anarthria—total loss of speech. Hemiparesis—one-sided muscle weakness that can affect your face, chest, arms, legs, or feet. Ataxia—loss of voluntary muscle control that may affect balance, co-ordination, and speech. Stridor – noisy breathing due to obstructed airflow in a blocked airway. Gross Haematuria—visible blood in urine. Infarcts—tissue death due to inadequate blood supply. Dysphagia—difficulty in swallowing.

I felt every piece of information a dawning. There was a precise word for the condition I was feeling—words I was hearing for the first time. It was an education.

My clinical abstract read: 'On the first hospital day, patient developed left sided weakness, facial asymmetry and onset of chills and heaviness of chest and headache . . .' Upon transfer to a sister hospital's ICU, my file read:

> Patient was received in the special unit with the above physical examination findings. However few hours later patient developed chills associated with worsening of dysarthria. Words were now incomprehensible and eventually this progressed to inability to move the right side of her body, with motor strength decreasing to 0-1/5 from 5/5. Further weakness in swallowing was also noted . . . Nasogastric tube was then inserted . . . Saliva was suctioned accordingly . . . Patient also had frequent coughing along with desaturation to 92% at room air hence

given O^2 support at 2LPM via nasal cannula . . . Condition was explained to family. Patient was then referred to pulmonary, with impression of aspiration pneumonia . . . FBC was inserted since patient was not able to spontaneously void. Hospital Day 2 (March 24) . . . Patient developed stridor. Nebulization, Cough-Assist Device, and Chest Physiotherapy were initiated. Eventually patient was hooked to BIPAP and referred to ENT for evaluation and to rule out possible vocal cord analysis [sic] . . . Hospital Day 3-4 . . . Enoxaparin was placed on hold due to gross hematuria . . . Hospital Day 8 . . . No signs of Retinal Vasculitis noted.[15] . . . However, on the 15th hospital day, patient noted recurrence of the left upper extremity tingling/pins and needles sensation associated with chest tightness, which was noted to be similar to her first presentation of stroke. Vital signs were stable. Thus repeat MRI plain of the brain was done which showed the previously noted infarct in the right medulla and left pons. Over the day, the symptom remained and was not progressive nor evolving. MRI was repeated the following day, now showing a tiny 3 MM acute infarct in the lateral aspect of the left medulla, with stable infarcts in the right medulla and left pons . . . Patient was referred to ID service for clearance prior to starting Rituximab. Blood, urine, and repeat sputum cultures were taken . . . Sputum gene expert did not detect any MTB. However, repeat sputum culture eventually showed of pseudomonas aeruginosa . . . Rituximab was placed on hold . . . Patient was cleared for travel via air ambulance by all co-managing services.

I felt like I was watching a fast-paced thriller. I was a rambling mess of medical jargon. Now, I was privy to what the doctors were reading outside my window. Medical and technical terms discussed outside my window seemed to objectify and blur the

---

[15] I seemed to have shown progress from Day 8.

humanity inside my room. My mom hardly wanted to go out, not wanting to hear the fate that befell me.

My lawyer brain quickly ferreted what didn't seem to make sense out of the hospital narrative. I didn't develop left side weakness on my first hospital day. I fumbled out of the car to the emergency room. My left-hand side was already weak when I climbed down the stairs of our home to rush to the hospital. I felt pins and needles leading to muscle weakness on my left side *before* I went to the hospital. If they didn't catch that, I didn't know what they were taking down notes for. Twice, repeat MRIs had to be taken to reveal new infarcts. I remember we were relieved to belatedly find that the hospital was mandated to perform a procedure by the phrase, 'patient's order'. I remember asking for a CT scan several times from the resident, but I didn't know those exact two words. It took incredible energy and precious (wasted) time to request for a brain scan in the emergency room. One had to beg, argue, or twist an arm to get one. I reminded myself as I was getting hyped up reading my files that I couldn't rewind time and retrieve my normal self by launching a case. *It was not like people did not want me to get well. No one perhaps could have borne ill-motivations. You get what you get. My case could have happened to anyone.* I found myself giving myself a sobering talk every time vengeful feelings started to rise within me. For the first time, I understood not to devote my energies to so much strife and make it a reactionary slave to my anger, no matter how fair it felt. I always wanted to meet the intern or resident who received me in the emergency room that fateful night. I wanted her to see me crippled. I imagined the look on her face. I wanted the storm of my deficit to overtake her. I knew it was not her fault, but I wanted it so desperately to be. I wanted a fall guy. I thought seeing her would bring me closure, but it turned out reading my file was enough. So many people were trying to save me. It takes a village, as they say. They tried to save me more than anything. That was enough.

I was discharged with the following diagnoses and co-morbidities: 1) acute cerebrovascular disease infarct, right medulla, left medulla, and left pons, 2) To consider central nervous system vasculitis probably secondary to connective tissue disease (rheumatoid arthritis), 3) aspiration pneumonia (Klebsiella pneumoniae), 4) Hospital acquired pneumonia (Pseudomonas aeruginosa). I didn't even know I had aspiration pneumonia. I was extremely paranoid of getting it, unaware that I had gone through the thick of it. I had nine doctors attending to me, one for almost every organ of my body. I had twenty-six prescribed medications:

Levofloxacin, 1 tablet per NGT once a day 10 a.m.; Hydrochloroquine, 1 tablet per NGT once a day 6 a.m.; Prednisone, 1 tablet per NGT twice a day 6 a.m. – 6 p.m.; Azathioprine, 1 tablet per NGT twice a day 6 a.m. – 6 p.m.; Enoxaparin Sodium, 1 pre-filled syringe administered subcutaneously every 24 hours at 2 p.m.; Aspirin, 1 tablet per NGT once a day 6 a.m.; Clopidogrel, 1 tablet per NGT once a day 10 a.m.; Citicoline Sodium, every 6 hours; Atorvastatin, 1 tablet per NGT once a day 6 p.m.; Omeprazole, 1 capsule per NGT once a day 5 a.m.; Paracetamol, VIT. B1, B6, B12, 1 tablet per NGT once a day 6 a.m.; Folic Acid, 1 tablet per NGT once a day 10 a.m.; Cholecalciferolen [sic] Vitamin D3, 1 soft gel capsule per NGT once a day 10 a.m.; Calcium Carbonate, 1 tablet per NGT twice a day 10 a.m. – 10 p.m.; Carbohydrates, Fat, Protein, Fibre, Na, 1 sachet in 50 ml water per NGT once a day 6 p.m.; Betahistine DiHCL 1 tablet per NGT twice a day as needed for dizziness; Orphenadrine Citrate, Paracetamol, 1 tablet per NGT every 8 hours as needed for headache; Metoclopramide, 1 ampule IV every 8 hours as needed for nausea and vomiting; Ipratropium Salbutamol, 1 nebulae every 6 hours; Dextran 70, Hypromellose, 1 drop to left eye every 4 hours during waking hours; Chlorhexidine Gluconate, gargle with 10 ml 3 times a day; Anise Oil, Bergamot Oil, Extr. Chamomile, Cineole, Meth, spray unto oral mucosa every 6 hours or as needed for throat irritation; Mometasone Furoate, 1 spray per nostril twice a day 8 a.m. – 8 p.m.; Fat Solution, 1 ampule IN 30CC PNSS slow IV once a day; Sambucus Nigra, Primula Veris & Elatior, Rumex Crisp, 1 tablet per NGT thrice a day for 3 days; and Clonidine HCL, 1 tablet per NGT every 6 hours as needed for SBP greater than or equal to 180MMHG.

I was exhausted just reading them. The tediousness of their administration must have left me dry.

I arrived in Singapore thus: 'conscious, severe dysarthria, dysphagia (on nasogastric tube), very ataxic, unable to sit without support, requiring in dwelling urinary catheter, right hemiplegia, left facial palsy, left hemisensory loss.' My overall summary progress report read:

Acute dissection of the Vertebra-Basilar arteries resulting in complete paralysis of her right arm and leg, numbness and poor co-ordination in her right, inability to speak, swallow and urinate as well as persistent dizziness and generalized body discomfort and spasms. This was previously not diagnosed in Cebu hospital; she was instead treated with high-dose steroids for presumed vasculitis; complicated by recurrent urinary tract infections.

I was lost in the medical jargon, but this lit up in my brain: *This was previously not diagnosed in Cebu hospital.* The Singapore hospital noted that I first suffered acute symptoms on 22 March. If I wasn't admitted on 19 March due to a stroke, was I relatively treatable then? Did I, upon arrival at the ER, just have a transient ischemic attack—a stroke that lasts only a few minutes and leaves the patient relatively unimpaired? These questions, I was afraid, will remain open in my mind until I die.

I continued to leaf through my hospital files as if they were evidence for a case I had to sort through. There were folders of them. There were images of my body I couldn't understand. They seemed almost forensic, a body of knowledge I was totally ignorant of. I opened the Web and typed 'brainstem stroke'.

> A stroke occurs when blood supply to the brain is interrupted. The way a stroke affects the brain depends on which part of the brain suffers damage, and to what degree . . . Sitting just above the spinal cord, the brain stem controls your breathing, heartbeat, and blood pressure. It also controls your speech, swallowing, hearing, and eye movements . . . Impulses sent by other parts of the brain travel through the brain stem on their way to various body parts. We're dependent on brain stem function for survival. A brain stem stroke threatens vital bodily functions, making it a life-threatening condition.[16]

My stroke was like a plug being pulled out of socket; the appliance (my body) being cut off from its power source. The appliance was perfectly well, but it was off. *It affected my breathing.* What could be more basic and underpinning than breathing?

I continued to leaf through the folders. One contained my worksheets during out-patient speech therapy. One was of problem solving dated 26 May 2022. It read:

Q: What can you do with an old shirt besides wear it?
A: make it a canvas for artwork

Q: What can you do with a toothpick besides clean your teeth?
A: pin fruits

Q: What can you do with glue besides paste paper together
A: make slime

---

[16] Healthline. (n.d.). *Brain Stem Stroke.* https://www.healthline.com/health/brain-stem-stroke

Q: What can you do with a plastic milk container after it is empty?
A: make a vase of flowers

My handwriting scrawled large across the page. Another worksheet was for drawing conclusions. Dated 27 May 2022, it read:

Q: What can happen if you forget to water plants for a week?
A: they die

Q: What can happen if you do not lock your door when leaving home?
A: you can get broken in

Q: What can happen if you do not stop for a red light?
A: you can get into an accident

Q: What can happen if you do not pay your state taxes?
A: you can pay a penalty

I held postgraduate degrees, but I remember being exhilarated at the exercise. Finally, my brain was being used for something less elementary. Other patients were shown a spoon and did not have a clue what it was for. I had a lot of things to be thankful for.

I got to the bottom of the files. Kim had put in an envelope all the cards that I received in the hospital. I remembered my wall being plastered with myriads of them—some colourful, some funny, some intricate, some religious. I often wondered how the other rooms looked. Did they have cards to accompany them as well? A bare wall could be lonely company. Some of the letters seemed desperate to reach me. Some were addressed to me, 'a patient in the neurological ward.' Somehow the letters reached me, a testament to Singapore's postal system, a luxury compared to our postal system in the Philippines. I read the letters anew, now that I was relatively stable. Every day, I faced them in my hospital room, but never regarded them in the same way before. I guess when you are running a race, you don't really see your

cheerleaders until after the race. I closed the last card, with a
fluttery light feeling in my stomach.

Scenes from my time in the hospital started flashing in my
mind. I could see them very vividly. They played like a reel in my
mind. They were not even of significant events. They were of
mundane things, like manoeuvring to get into my pyjamas when
I could hardly move my legs; trying macaroni in tomato sauce
when I could just swallow; chatting with the nurses about how
understaffed they are; watching my family huddle every night to
share dinner; listening to the loud squawks of birds heralding
dusk in the city; going through the halls of the hospital and saying
hi to every random guard in their stations; just fishing for the
curious out of the ordinary. I lived through all those scenes again.
Amidst the grave events, there were the ordinary things that made
life still life.

I thought about Dr Lee and his two rabbits. Unbeknownst
to him, he had produced two rabbits under his hat. Maybe it was
never about the cure, but the eyes to see the silver lining in the
bleakest moment. Perhaps that is the greatest magic trick that
both doctor and patient have to work on: to see something out of
nothing. I am perhaps running on gratefulness, but it is an engine
I intend to run on my whole life.

I had a sweet and peaceful closure. The images in my brain
were no longer attended with trauma and heartache. Truly, joy
came with the morning.

Epilogue

They taught us *res gestae* in law school. Evidence that comes out just when an incident happens is likely to be true. A person cannot yet even think to fabricate a lie just after the heat of the moment.

I wrote shortly after discharge, just as my experience was unfolding before me. I wrote every day like I needed it. I wrote almost this entire book on paper with my left hand. Edward told me to start banking on my left while waiting for my right to regroup. My left was wobbly at best. My arm was like an unreliable crane. But I guess my will to write, to let out feelings to cure myself, was much greater. My penmanship evolved from what looked like chicken scratch to more legible handwriting. My notes bore nonsense until my brain found itself again and started forming sense. It astounds me until now how I managed to write so much. I was just writing for writing's sake.

When I got fairly better, I collected my journals and sat down to read them. Opening them was like unearthing a box of evidence. Each page told a story, a slice of my life as held frozen in time. There were things I wrote that was at the peak of what I could have learned at the time. As my recovery progressed, my learning became fuller. My wisdom matured in a way only time allowed. I'm glad I left room within myself for it to grow.

When I managed a few vignettes, I submitted my work to a publisher without any expectations. I had just begun what was to become my memoir. The publisher's website said that it would take at least six months for them to get back to me. By submitting,

I thought I had nothing to lose. But the next day, the publisher replied. It was neither a yes nor a no, but at least I got one foot in the door. I didn't hear from the publisher until months later, but I wrote with the assuredness of a woman with a book deal yet the freedom of a woman without. Later, a deal did materialize. I was thus the invalid with the coolest job.

My doctor said, quoting a Chinese proverb, that 'you write not because you have an answer to something but because you have a song.' There must have been something compulsive in my song. I remember forcing my very heavy left arm across the page to write what I needed. You don't need to know my qualms, how I think I managed to get the stroke. My words would matter to anyone who wants to know how I managed through my ordeal and what I thought about while I recovered. For sure, my qualms are many and complicated. It's the last thing on my mind to portray my life as perfect. If I told you each of them, then my story would be personal, when suffering is universal. I don't want to detract from that. By no means is my story ended; I will continue in convalescence. But everything I've written up to this point—it is all res gestae. Perhaps some need to stew a bit so as not to sound selfish, but it is all res gestae. I assume all proper recordal should be.

My stroke is like being given the chance to fast-forward through the tape of my life then to rewind it to live it more gracefully. No one now could tell me what I am made of. I know myself from suffering with such a definitiveness that I could not be budged. There is a deep security in that. I no longer feel like this balloon drifting endlessly higher and only getting smaller in the atmosphere until it disappears from view. On the contrary, I feel firmly tied to the hand of my Father that I could go anywhere and feel safe. It is an incredibly liberating feeling. I'd already arrived even before I set out. I'm tethered.

A Letter from Dr Lee:

Dear Tracy,

I can hardly remember the last time I wrote to anyone, let alone my patients. After all the countless boxes of OTAP biscuits, cards, words, books and gifts, I decided to add a few more lines to those loving anecdotes and silly quotes that you've already heard ad nauseam.

"Where are they?" Those words rang deep in my heart and mind when I read what you wrote in a note, wondering about the inner strength, peace and faith that you'll need so badly in your daily struggles. Indeed we all ask the same as pilgrims on the earth with our citizenship in God's kingdom. Yet, our "inheritance is imperishable, undefiled, and unfading," as promised in 1 Peter 1:4.

So press on, my dear patient, and hold no fear, no matter where you go and where you are.

> "When you remember me, it means you have carried something of who I am with you, that I have left some mark of who I am on who you are. It means that you can summon me back to your mind even though countless years and miles may stand between us. It means that if we meet again, you will know me."

Wishing you the abundant blessings of our LORD JESUS CHRIST as you journey onward!

Your doctor,
DR LEE KIM EN

29 NOV 2022
SINGAPORE

Dear Tracy,

I can hardly remember the last time
I wrote to anyone, let alone my patients
after all the countless boxes of OTAP
biscuits, cards, words, books & gifts.
I decided to add a few more lines
to those boring anecdotes & silly
quotes that you've already heard
ad nauseum.

"Where are they?" Those words rang
deep in my heart & mind when I
read what you wrote in a note,
wondering about the inner strength,
peace & faith that you'll need so
badly in your daily struggles. Indeed
we all ask the same as pilgrims on
the earth with our citizenship in
God's kingdom. Yet, our "inheritance
is imperishable, undefiled, and
unfading", as promised in 1 Pete 1:4.

So press on, my dear patient, and hold no fear, no matter where you go & where you are

"When you remember me, it means you have carried something of who I am with you, that I have left some mark of who I am on who you are. It means that you can summon me back to your mind even though countless years and miles may stand between us. It means that if we meet again, you will know me."

Wishing you the abundant blessings of our LORD JESUS CHRIST as you journey onward!

Your doctor,

DR LEE KIM EN.

Letter by Dr Lee. Quote in the letter is by Frederick Buechner.

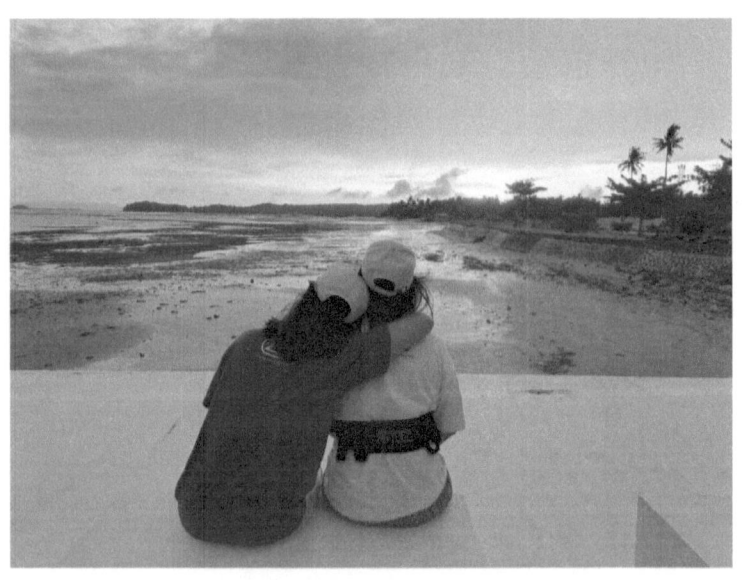

Catching sunrise with Kim

Acknowledgements

'When you pass through the waters, I will be with you.'[17] I got to live through that promise. Thank you, Jesus. Your love will not let me go.

To my family—James, Annie, Kim, and Mimi—no one could have borne my experience like you did. Thank you, and I love you.

To my aunts and uncles, Jan and Ed, Jun and Victoria, Sanilhyn, Baby and Romy, Libeth and Judy, Mila, Jaime and Angie, James—you took up my cause like it was yours. Thank you.

To my guardian angel, my grandmother Adelina, this book and Blithe Books are for you.

To Lola, I now know what you went through in the hospital. Thank you for keeping me company.

To Mama Lenny, who would have known that the daily prayers I attended for you would eventually include me too? A special thank you to my loving Hill and King families. I survived because of your prayers.

To my devoted Aunt Jan for editing my writing multiple times, for Mimi for fact-checking my memory of my time in the hospital, to Mom and Jacques for helping me type my handwritten manuscript, thank you for your invaluable help.

To Drs Lee, Lui, and Wee, I can't be under better care. To Sandra, Cindy, and Lily—I actually miss going to your clinic.

---

[17] Isaiah 43:2

To Drs Jeremy Lim and Karen Chua, thank you very much for leading me to Dr Lee when it would have been convenient to dismiss me.

To all my Singapore nurses, particularly Zoraida, Jesse, Sue, Christina, Ban-Ban, Nalina, Irene, Glenda, KK, Bella, Nur, Guy, Goki, Arasi, Glyza, Mohammed, Liz, you made the hospital home.

To Edward, Hui Shi, Hui Yong, Hui Jun, Pam, JK, Han, Yvonne, Avi, Mary, Mama Cat, Siva, Belle, William, Zul, Christina, Vini, Irene, Colleen, Andrew, Yu Hui, Tyler, Nat, Jolene Johan, John, Cory, Sima, and the rest of my rehab family, you made rehab the coolest place to hang out.

To all my Philippine doctors and sweet nurses (Laura and her team), thank you.

To my Singapore family—Henry, Sajeda and Naweed, Mickael, Stef, James, Giulia, Emma, Devan, Vince, Vickneshvaran, Sasitharan, Glenn, Vijay, Kamala, Mr. Lim, Mr. Ong, YiYang and Michael, Papa Santos, Mama Yennie, Uncle Bernard and Auntie Mae, you made the months I spent there charming.

To my classmates in rehab, thank you for teaching me for life.

To the Kandaya staff, you ease me into life; To Ezra, you show me what life is all about. To my birthday architects, Louie and Annette, I didn't expect the fireworks.

To Liv, Jing, and Shammy, thank you for always urging me to write.

To Earla, Jances, Gay, Regie, RJ, Abby, Ciela, I had your cards in my room in Singapore. To Sky, for the loving notes.

To my friends, I am loath to mention names lest I forget anyone by mistake, thank you for your thoughtfulness.

To my prayer warriors—Aunties and Uncles Vicky, Rose and Henry, Grace and Justo, Pinky, June, Lilibeth, Dr Mitz, Jenny, Gina, Jack and Rita, Eliseo and Genelou, Edwin and Joy, Romy and Evelyn, Richard and Ellen, Em-em, Cathy, Alvin,

Carlson, Arlene, Gus and Edith, Dr Rowena, Tess and Joseph, Kerwin and Virgie, Jimson and Grace, Orman, Dani, Pammy and Lolong and family, Jun and Cynthia, Mae, George, Irene, Stephanie, Pelsie, Alex and Alma, Eddie and Sylvia, Rosita; Sr Regie, Fr Rustia, Pastor Pat, Trappestine Sisters, Dr Mitz' Bible Study group, Ptr. Steve and Marg; Alex, Ana and Wesley, Coleen; Hannah; my cousins from both sides, LVL, MMM, Ms Mao, Ms Josie; Hannah; Fiesta Appliance employees, thank you for keeping me in your prayers.

To Uncles and Aunties Boy, Anita, Hans, Tong-Cheng who make a pit stop to visit me every time they're in Cebu, thank you.

To Christopher, Alyssa, and Lance, you are family in Cebu; Thank you for being willing accomplices to my recovery.

To Uncles and Aunties Joy and Edwin, Boy and Jean; Shannon, Tim, Uncle Edward, Nicole, Jamie, Kimmee, Agnes, thanks for your invaluable help.

To Mickie, my ever-reliable insurance agent and friend, you were unwavering at the critical times, and that has made all the difference.

To my understanding clients and friends, Michelle and Christian, and to my UC Law family, thank you for making everything easy for me when I needed it to be.

To Ailyn, Ann, Jay-Ann, for holding the fort while we were away; to Kim, Joy, and Analee, for helping with Blithe while I was incapacitated.

To Mai-Mai, for caring for me at my critical moments, and for Mae for ably following suit, thank you from the bottom of my heart.

To Sandy Daza, thank you for making my day in the hospital.

To the team of PRH SEA, particularly Nora, Swadha, Thatchaa, and Divya, thank you for making it happen for me.

To my Blithe Books readers, I hold you in my heart.

'But those who hope in the LORD will renew their strength. They will soar on wings like eagles; they will run and not grow weary, they will walk and not be faint.'

—Isaiah 40:31, NIV